HIV and Community
Mental Healthcare

HIV and Community Mental Healthcare

Edited by

Michael D. Knox and

Caroline H. Sparks

The Johns Hopkins University Press

Baltimore and London

Printed in the United States of America on acid-free paper

07 06 05 04 03 02 01 00 99 98 5 4 3 2 1

The Johns Hopkins University Press
2715 North Charles Street
Baltimore, Maryland 21218-4319

The Johns Hopkins University Press Ltd., London

Library of Congress Cataloging-in-Publication Data

HIV and community mental healthcare/edited by Michael D. Knox, Caroline H. Sparks.
   p. cm.
Includes bibliographical references and index.
ISBN 0-8018-5803-8 (alk. paper)—ISBN 0-8018-5084-6 (pbk. : alk. paper)
  1. AIDS (Disease)—Psychological aspects. 2. Community mental health services.
I. Knox, Michael D. II. Sparks, Caroline H. (Caroline Heyward)
  [DNLM: 1. HIV Infections—psychology. 2. HIV Infections—psychology—programmed
instruction. 3. Mental Disorders—therapy. 4. Mental Disorders—therapy—
programmed instruction. 5. Community Mental Health Services—organization &
administration. 6. Attitude of Health Personnel. WC 503.2 H6764 1998]
RC607.A26H5688 1998
362. 1'969792'0019—dc21
DNLM/DLC
for Library of Congress   97-24462   CIP

A catalog record for this book is available from the British Library.

Contents

II

Understanding HIV Healthcare

III

Mental Health Interventions for HIV

III

Special Topics

Preface

We created *HIV and Community Mental Healthcare* for clinical and management staff of community mental health centers (CMHCs) and other public mental health programs and for upper-level undergraduate students and graduate students in psychology, social work, mental health nursing, counseling, public health, psychiatry, and other fields related to health and mental health. It is intended to help this audience improve their ability to care for persons affected by HIV and AIDS.

The text is organized into four sections: The Challenge of HIV for Community Mental Health, Understanding HIV Healthcare, Mental Health Interventions for HIV, and Special Topics. This is the first book to focus on the unique contributions to prevention and treatment that community mental health workers may make by providing appropriate services to persons affected by HIV.

Since the first AIDS cases were identified, we have learned much about the disease and its treatment. HIV-infected persons experience a wide range of psychological and neuropsychological problems that may require mental health treatment. Their family, friends, and healthcare workers may also need mental health services. In addition, people who are at risk of infection because of life-style may also benefit from sensitive community mental health interventions.

Community mental health centers are uniquely positioned to provide vital mental health services to individuals, families, and communities affected by the HIV epidemic. One barrier to the provision of these services by CMHC staff is a lack of knowledge and skills needed to assist these persons. It is our hope that this book will help workers and students to improve their understanding of HIV and to develop or improve their capabilities to deliver HIV-related mental healthcare.

Researchers, teachers, and practitioners with demonstrated leadership in community mental healthcare pertaining to HIV contributed to this book by writing about their specific areas of expertise. We have included topics that address the provision of appropriate mental health interventions for individual clients, their families, friends, and the community.

We want this book to accomplish four major goals. First, it should help increase the ability of CMHC staff and students in the field to identify the HIV-related needs of their clients and to deliver more effective services. Second, since there is evidence that some CMHC staff avoid interacting with persons with HIV disease, the book is intended to increase their comfort level and sensitivity. Third, the book seeks to increase staff knowledge about HIV-related signs and symptoms so that clinicians who provide care may conduct adequate screening and make appropriate referrals. Understanding the disease, its diagnosis, and treatment will improve communication with other healthcare workers and increase understanding of the experiences of infected clients. Fourth, the text provides accurate and up-to-date information about HIV disease that should allow CMHC staff to assist their communities in overcoming the fear and anxiety often associated with HIV/AIDS.

HIV and Community Mental Healthcare may be read in its entirety or selected chapters may be used for in-service training or university courses. Each chapter's text is preceded by learning objectives and an outline. Review questions, references, and suggested readings are included at the end of each chapter. The appendix is a comprehensive directory of HIV/AIDS resources.

Acknowledgments

The editors thank the authors of each chapter for contributing their expertise to the development of this text. It has been a pleasure to have the opportunity to interact with persons around the country who are knowledgeable about HIV and community mental health.

Some of the content of this book is based, in part, on training materials initially developed by the authors to fulfill National Institute of Mental Health (NIMH) professional service contract number 91MFO8211601D issued to the National Council of Community Mental Health Centers. Please note that the views expressed in this book are those of the authors and do not necessarily reflect the official position of the NIMH, the National Community Mental Healthcare Council (NCMHC), or the University of South Florida.

For their support and encouragement, our special thanks and appreciation go to Charles G. Ray, Chief Executive Officer of the NCMHC; Juan Ramos, Ph.D., and Armand Checker, M.S., of the NIMH; and Max C. Dertke, Ph.D., former Dean, David L. Shern, Ph.D., Dean of the Louis de la Parte Florida Mental Health Institute (FMHI), University of South Florida, and Gregory B. Teague, Ph.D., Chair of the Department of Community Mental Health, FMHI.

Assistance has been provided by many faculty and staff of the Department of Community Mental Health at FMHI and the University of South Florida's Center for HIV Education and Research (which is funded, in part, by the Health Resources and Services Administration grant DHHS-BHP 2U69 PE00101-07). Special acknowledgment is extended to Jason M. Longo, M.A., and Kelly M. Lyon, B.I.S., for coordinating this project. We thank Charles F. Clark, M.D.; Martha A. Friedrich, Ph.D.; Pam McGlinchey, M.A., M.P.H.; Lucinda P. Knox, M.S.W.;

Michael W. Sharinus, Ph.D.; John A. Grannan, M.A.; and John Martin, Ph.D., for their consultation, factual reviews, and proofreading of chapters, and Christine Smith for providing clerical support. We also express gratitude to Ardis Hanson, M.A., Leslie Chason, M.A., and Walter Cone, M.L.A., of the FMHI Library, who have always been available to assist in locating and verifying references for each chapter.

We express our appreciation to the following people for their assistance on this project: Wendy Harris, medical editor; Barbara B. Lamb, managing editor; and Dana Battaglia, production coordinator of the Johns Hopkins University Press, and Anne Stewart Seitz of York Production Services.

List of Contributors

Timothy L. Boaz, Ph.D., Associate Professor, Department of Community Mental Health, Louis de la Parte Florida Mental Health Institute, University of South Florida, Tampa, Florida.

Nicolás P. Carballeira, N.D., M.P.H., Director and Chief Executive Officer, Latino Health Institute of Massachusetts, and Lecturer, Boston University School of Public Health, Boston, Massachusetts.

Frank Chessa, M.A., Lecturer, Department of Philosophy, Georgetown University, Washington, D.C.

Charles F. Clark, M.D., M.P.H., Visiting Associate Professor, Department of Community Mental Health, Louis de la Parte Florida Mental Health Institute, University of South Florida, Tampa, Florida; and Psychiatrist, Jefferson Center for Mental Health, Arvada, Colorado.

Michael G. Dow, Ph.D., Professor and Director of Research, Department of Community Mental Health, Louis de la Parte Florida Mental Health Institute, University of South Florida, Tampa, Florida.

Martha A. Friedrich, Ph.D., Clinical Assistant Professor, Department of

Community Mental Health, Louis de la Parte Florida Mental Health Institute, University of South Florida, Tampa, Florida.

Jeremy S. Gaies, Psy.D., Psychologist in private practice; former Clinical Assistant Professor, Department of Community Mental Health, Louis de la Parte Florida Mental Health Institute, University of South Florida, Tampa, Florida.

John A. Grannan, M.A., Senior Training Specialist, Center for HIV Education and Research, Louis de la Parte Florida Mental Health Institute, University of South Florida, Tampa, Florida.

Mary Kay Houston-Vega, Ph.D., M.S.W., Associate Professor, School of Social Work, Barry University, Miami, Florida.

Michael D. Knox, Ph.D., Distinguished Service Professor; Professor, Department of Community Mental Health, Louis de la Parte Florida Mental Health Institute; Professor of Medicine, Department of Internal Medicine; Director, USF Center for HIV Education and Research, University of South Florida, Tampa, Florida. He is a licensed psychologist who received his Ph.D. in community psychology in 1974 from the University of Michigan.

Joline Miceli-Mullen, J.D., Visiting Assistant Professor, Department of Community Mental Health, Louis de la Parte Florida Mental Health Institute, University of South Florida; and Vice President Legal Services, University Community Hospital, Tampa, Florida.

Kathleen Miner, Ph.D., M.P.H., Associate Dean for Applied Public Health and Associate Professor, Department of Behavioral Sciences and Health Education, Rollins School of Public Health, Emory University, Atlanta, Georgia.

Rubén Montano-López, M.A., Department of Family Services, Brookside Community Health Center, Brigham and Women's Hospital, Boston, Massachusetts.

Robert P. Nelson, Jr., M.D., Associate Professor of Medicine and Pediatrics,

University of South Florida College of Medicine; and Visiting Associate Professor, Department of Community Mental Health, Louis de la Parte Florida Mental Health Institute, University of South Florida, Tampa, Florida.

José A. Parés-Avila, M.A., Department of Mental Health and Addictions, Fenway Community Health Center; and Department of Psychiatry, Harvard Medical School, Boston, Massachusetts.

Barbara Russell, R.N., C.I.C., A.C.R.N., M.P.H., Visiting Instructor, Department of Community Mental Health, Louis de la Parte Florida Mental Health Institute, University of South Florida, Tampa; and Director of Infection Control, Baptist Hospital, Miami, Florida.

Caroline H. Sparks, Ph.D., Assistant Research Professor, Department of Prevention and Community Health, School of Public Health, and Fellow of the Institute for Health Policy, Outcomes and Human Values, George Washington University, Washington, D.C. She is a licensed psychologist who received her Ph.D. in psychology from The Ohio State University in 1979.

Derise E. Tolliver, Ph.D., Assistant Professor, School for New Learning, DePaul University, Chicago, Illinois; and AIDS Education Consultant, National Association of Black Psychologists, Washington, D.C.

Robert M. Walker, M.D., Director, Division of Medical Ethics and Humanities; and Associate Professor, Department of Internal Medicine, University of South Florida College of Medicine, Tampa, Florida.

John C. Ward, Jr., Ph.D., Associate Professor and Associate Chair, Department of Community Mental Health, Louis de la Parte Florida Mental Health Institute, University of South Florida, Tampa, Florida.

Mark G. Winiarski, Ph.D., Director, AIDS Mental Health and Primary Care Integration Project, Montefiore Medical Center; and Assistant Professor, Departments of Family Medicine and Psychiatry, Albert Einstein College of Medicine, Bronx, New York.

Part I

The Challenge of HIV for Community Mental Health

Chapter 1

HIV-Related Community Mental Health Services

Michael D. Knox, Ph.D.

Overview

This chapter demonstrates the need for a broad range of HIV-related community mental health services and introduces the reader to the patients and clients who are in need of these services. Clinicians and administrators will be made more aware of the magnitude and scope of the AIDS crisis from the perspective of community mental health. This chapter draws on work by Knox, M.D., Davis, M., & Friedrich, M.A. (1994), published in *Community Mental Health Journal.*

Learning Objectives

1. To identify common psychological stressors associated with HIV infection.

2. To identify common mental health problems associated with HIV infection.

3. To recognize populations of potential clients who may be in need of community mental health services related to HIV/AIDS.

4. To understand specialized HIV-related services that can be provided by community mental health centers.

5. To recognize the importance of staff attitudes and knowledge in the care of persons with HIV-related conditions.

Outline

I. The HIV Mental Health Challenge
   A. Need for mental health services
   B. Common psychological stressors faced by HIV-infected persons
   C. Common mental health problems associated with HIV infection

II. HIV Mental Health Service Needs
   A. The HIV mental health spectrum
   B. Services to those who are not infected
      1. General community
      2. Healthcare workers
      3. Family members and significant others
      4. Persons engaging in unsafe behavior
   C. Services to persons with HIV disease
      1. Persons who are HIV-infected (asymptomatic)
      2. Persons experiencing early disease manifestations
      3. Persons with AIDS

III. Staff Knowledge and Attitudes

IV. Conclusion

The HIV Mental Health Challenge

The HIV epidemic is generating an enormous need for mental health services. The deadly nature of the infection, the behaviors that facilitate transmission, the interaction between psychological well-being and immune system functioning, the occurrence of dementia, and the stress placed on family, friends, and caregivers have created a challenge of staggering proportions for community mental health. Mental health professionals should play a central role in AIDS education, prevention, and treatment.

On any given day, there are more people in need of HIV-related community mental healthcare than there are people requiring HIV-related medical care. The epidemic is having profound psychological effects not only on those infected but also on their families and the communities in which they live. Mental healthcare can change attitudes and behaviors and help reduce the spread of HIV. For those who are already infected, mental health treatment can have a significant positive impact on the quality and length of life. The field of community mental health has not yet recognized the magnitude of the situation. Most clinicians are not prepared to provide the broad range of specialized services that are needed. Community mental health providers must be trained for their role in the HIV crisis.

Special characteristics of this disease contribute to its adverse psychological impact. Stressors result from feelings of guilt, pain, weakness, the progressive course of the disease, and medical complications. Social ostracism and discrimination compound the emotional trauma of HIV disease. The following list identifies common psychological stressors faced by persons with HIV infection.

Common Psychological Stressors Faced by HIV-Infected Persons

- Social isolation and stigmatization
- Public revelation of sexual orientation or drug use
- Estrangement from family
- Death of friends from AIDS
- Loss of job, housing, insurance, savings, etc.
- Sexual conflicts—inhibition or unsafe sex
- Guilt over life-style and past behaviors
- Loss of physical and mental abilities
- Dependency and loss of autonomy
- Pain and disfigurement
- Chronic fatigue and weakness
- Uncertainty about disease progression
- Infections and sickness
- Likelihood of an early death

Psychological stress may have a negative effect on a person's immune system and have consequences for how rapidly symptoms develop. For persons with AIDS, an intense stress reaction may lead to greater vulnerability of infection.

Typical mental dysfunctions associated with HIV disease are depression, anxiety disorders, adjustment disorders, suicidal crisis, panic disorder, exacerbation of pre-existing mental illness, and drug and alcohol abuse. Additionally, HIV frequently attacks the central nervous system, producing problems with memory, motivation, and intellectual functioning. Serious and debilitating neuropsychological symptoms may make patient care difficult for health professionals and frightening for family and friends.

Common Mental Health Problems Associated with HIV Infection

- Depression
- Anxiety disorders
- Adjustment disorders
- Suicidal crises
- Panic disorder
- Exacerbation of pre-existing mental illness
- Drug and alcohol abuse
- Organic mental disorders

With neither cure nor vaccine likely to be available soon, the only way to reduce the spread of HIV is to promote safer sexual and drug-using practices among those infected and those at risk. In addition, behavioral interventions such as stress management, relaxation training, and exercise may provide considerable benefit to immune functioning and improve psychological well-being. (See Chapter 11, "Effects of Stress: The Relationship between Health and Stress.") Mental health professionals should play a central role in AIDS education, prevention, and treatment.

Many community mental health centers (CMHCs) and other public and private mental health agencies are unprepared to meet the challenges of the HIV epidemic and to provide for the needs of persons with HIV-related conditions. Funding for HIV-related mental health programs is almost nonexistent. Many CMHC staff lack the necessary skills and knowledge or feel uncomfortable treating HIV-infected clients. There is a need for ongoing continuing education of mental health providers about HIV to increase knowledge, improve clinical skills, modify attitudes, and reduce discomfort. A broad spectrum of mental health services is needed and must become more widely recognized and available.

Clinicians must be able to recognize and understand the cognitive, behavioral, and emotional concomitants of the HIV epidemic. They should be prepared to offer services to people during all stages of the illness. This array of AIDS-related services must be broad both in terms of the individuals to be served and the specialized services to be provided. As the epidemic grows, the number of those affected, directly and indirectly, will produce increasing demands for effective community mental healthcare.

HIV Mental Health Service Needs

Community mental healthcare is responsible for providing services needed by all people affected by this disease, whether infected by the virus or not. Populations in need of community mental health services include the general community, healthcare workers, persons engaging in unsafe behaviors, HIV-infected persons, those with AIDS, and the families, friends, and significant others of infected persons.

The HIV Mental Health Spectrum

The HIV mental health spectrum identifies the service needs for a broad population of potential clients. This model represents the people affected by AIDS who may be in need of psychological interventions.

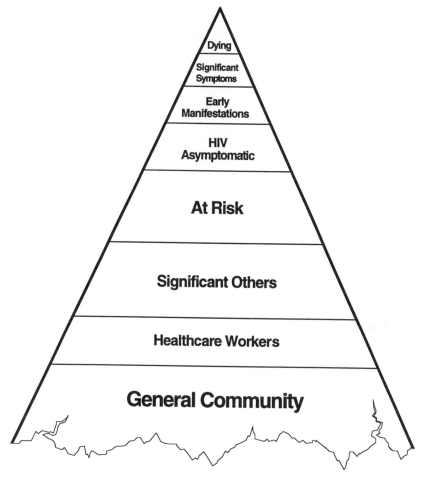

FIGURE 1.1 The HIV Mental Health Spectrum-Persons Affected by AIDS
Adapted from Knox, M.D., Davis, M., & Friedrich, M.A. (1994).

The lower portion of the figure, including its base, represents noninfected members of the general population who are psychologically affected by this disease. Above the base, the psychological impact of HIV becomes more direct. HIV-infected persons, whether or not they are experiencing symptoms, constitute the upper third of the figure. Moving up the spectrum pyramid, the symptomatology and the need for medical and psychological services increases.

Services to Those Who Are Not Infected

Many people still believe that they are not affected by HIV because they are not infected, do not know anyone who is infected, and do not recognize their risk of becoming infected. With increasing cost to government and business, with the strains HIV places on our overburdened healthcare system, and with the risks it imposes on sexually active persons, everyone is affected by HIV.

All people need accurate information about HIV and its transmission. This should lead to safer health and personal practices and to increased awareness of the social implications of the epidemic. A failure to provide appropriate information will likely lead to a wider and more rapid spread of the disease and unnecessary suffering by those who are infected, as well as by their friends, families, and communities.

Services to the General Community

- Consultation and collaboration with public health and other healthcare workers
- Educational programs designed to change behavior and attitudes

The human immunodeficiency virus is transmitted by specific individual human behaviors. To be effective, medical and public health interventions must include psychological and behavioral perspectives. Although considerable educational efforts to teach the public about HIV have been made, irrational fears, prejudice, and unsafe behaviors persist. Community mental health providers should play an important role in campaigns to reduce prejudice and fear, to promote accurate knowledge, and to facilitate behavioral change. These professionals should support and enhance public health efforts aimed at HIV-related education, prevention, and attitude change. Consultation and collaboration with public health and other healthcare workers are important CMHC services.

Most adolescents and adults know the principal modes of HIV transmission. Nonetheless, misconceptions about transmission through casual contact are common, lead to heightened anxiety about risk of infection, and may lead to discrimination against those who are infected. Thus, CMHCs should offer educational programs designed to change behavior and attitudes.

Services to Healthcare Workers

- Support groups for healthcare providers
- Individual and family psychotherapy
- Stress management programs

Clinicians can assist healthcare providers to examine their feelings about working with individuals infected with HIV and to improve their comfort and effectiveness in treating these patients. Community mental health centers may offer support groups for healthcare providers that can be critical for helping to prevent burnout. Such groups also allow for the sharing of information and the identification of relevant community resources. Centers can also provide individual and family psychotherapy to help reduce biases and fears, as well as offer stress management programs especially geared toward the healthcare provider.

Services to Family Members and Significant Others

- Support groups
- Crisis intervention
- Family/couples psychotherapy
- Bereavement counseling
- Children's services
- Training to provide cognitive stimulation and to maximize mental functioning and self-care

Family members and significant others face many emotional challenges and can benefit from a wide range of services from support groups and crisis intervention to family/couples psychotherapy and bereavement counseling. The needs and numbers of affected families are growing rapidly. Loved ones often provide the main source of emotional support for a person with AIDS. While providing care, they must also cope with their own fears, their anticipated loss, and finally, their grief.

Significant others and family members may need to deal with additional family conflict as a result of facing AIDS. Often, previously kept secrets regarding sexual or drug use behavior are disclosed at the same time as the AIDS diagnosis. This further complicates the family's response. Conflicts often arise between families of origin and current sexual partners. Family therapy and multiple family groups can be effective in resolving or reducing these conflicts.

Children of persons with AIDS face a different set of challenges because of their immaturity and dependence on caretakers. They must cope with anxiety produced by their parents' emotional struggles related to the illness, reduced predictability of their environment, anticipation of parental loss, and eventually, grief for the lost parent.

Children must often face previously unknown aspects of a parent's life-style and cope with changing caretakers. When the AIDS patient is a child, clinicians must consider the developmental stage of the child while helping him or her cope with fears of illness, treatment, and death. Parents of children with AIDS generally have intense feelings of helplessness, guilt, and depression. This is particularly true if the child was infected during fetal development, delivery, or breast-feeding. Many issues must also be considered when helping a child face the loss of a sibling to AIDS. Community mental health centers should offer specialized children's services that are attuned to the challenges faced by children and their families.

Clinicians can help family members and friends to understand and to cope with AIDS-related dementia and its wrenching consequences. Caregivers should be instructed about dementia so that they can understand the patient's behavior. Caregivers can be trained to provide cognitive stimulation to maximize mental functioning and sustain self-care.

Services to Persons Engaging in Risky Behavior

- HIV/AIDS education
- Safer sex education
- Training in communication and assertiveness skills
- Substance abuse treatment programs
- Individual psychotherapy

Mental health professionals are aware that accurate knowledge does not necessarily lead to safer behavior. Many people still use condoms infrequently despite widespread knowledge of their effectiveness in preventing HIV transmission. For many, even discussing AIDS with one's sexual partner is a rare occurrence.

People often underestimate their own risk of infection, thereby reducing the probability of their taking preventive measures. It is imperative that educational programs include efforts to produce attitudinal and behavioral change in addition to increased knowledge.

Community mental health centers must also develop services that are tailored to the risks most likely to affect their current clients. Clients often cope by denying their risk. This denial may prevent clients from believing that the information is relevant to their situation. Others may acknowledge their risk status but experience anxiety that interferes with learning. Services aimed at AIDS risk reduction should include techniques to reduce both denial and anxiety.

Client HIV/AIDS education must include current information, especially regarding modes of transmission. Safer sex techniques must be explained, and condom use must be taught with opportunities for practice. It is important that individuals learn the behaviors needed to avoid transmission and that they be desensitized to the anxiety associated with changing their sexual practices. (See Chapter 17, "Treating Persons with Serious and Persistent Mental Illness.")

Communication and assertiveness skills development are an essential part of learning to reduce risk. Substance abuse treatment programs and individual psychotherapy also help people who are not yet infected, but who have difficulty changing behaviors that put them at risk.

Drug and alcohol use increase HIV transmission risk by several mechanisms. Intoxication can lower sexual inhibitions and increase impulsive behavior, which makes it difficult to employ HIV prevention techniques. Sex-for-drugs transactions may accompany drug use and are unlikely to be associated with the use of condoms. The immunosuppressive effects of drugs may increase the likelihood of HIV infection and accelerate the development of symptoms.

Injecting drug use is risky because of the common practice of sharing needles and paraphernalia. It is one of the major modes of HIV transmission. Although elimination of drug use is the focus of many treatment plans, this must be balanced with efforts to teach needle and paraphernalia cleaning techniques or replacement while an individual is still using drugs. It is clear that drug use does lead to increased risk of HIV infection by a variety of mechanisms. (See Chapter 18, "Treating Persons Who Use Drugs.")

Additionally, some individuals may need extensive counseling to overcome anxieties about being tested for HIV. Clinicians need to address concerns about anonymity and confidentiality, emphasize the importance of early detection, and help plan what to do in the event of a positive test result. The importance of this pre-test counseling is even greater with the availability of home-testing.

Persons with chronic and severe mental illness may be at increased risk of contracting HIV. In some areas of the United States, 5–20 percent of persons admitted to private and public mental health facilities are reported to test positive for HIV antibodies. Low-functioning clients with poor interpersonal skills, who lack resources and social support systems, will be especially difficult to treat. New approaches need to be developed to work with these clients to prevent further spread of the virus and to deal with the additional stress placed on already fragile psyches. In addition, clinicians can play an important role in the early detection of HIV infection among their clients. (See Chapter 5, "The Clinician's Role in Early Detection of HIV.")

Services to Persons with HIV Disease

Mental health interventions for those with diagnosed HIV infection, whether asymptomatic or ill, may include crisis intervention, suicide risk assessment, supportive counseling, psychotherapy, support groups, neuropsychological assessment, and memory enhancement training. These are traditional clinical services that must be offered by trained staff with specialized knowledge of HIV. Listed below are a variety of services that CMHCs can make available to HIV-infected persons.

Services for Persons with HIV Disease

- Crisis intervention
- Psychological evaluation
- Suicide risk assessment
- Supportive counseling
- Psychotherapy
- Support groups
- Neuropsychological assessment
- Memory enhancement training
- Training in health enhancing behaviors
- Stress management
- Relaxation training, hypnosis, and imagery
- Family therapy
- Case management services

- Recreational and occupational therapy
- Psychotropic medications
- Day treatment
- Hospice care
- Death and dying therapy

Individuals with HIV infection who have not yet developed AIDS can benefit from community mental health services that help reduce stress, change behavior, aid life planning, help cope with guilt feelings, and treat depression. Behavior change is necessary to avoid reinfection and infecting others. Training in health-enhancing behavior such as adequate nutrition, rest, exercise, and avoidance and reduction of stress and drug use may help to slow the decline of the immune system. Stress management protocols, including relaxation training, hypnosis, and imagery, can be of great benefit.

Psychological interventions should be a critical part of the treatment of HIV infection. Learning that one is HIV-infected can produce a variety of emotions, including: anger, guilt, helplessness, sadness, loneliness, hopelessness, and anxiety. It may also result in disclosure of sexual or drug use behavior that the individual would have preferred to keep secret. Anxiety disorders and depression may result in suicide attempts, social isolation, increased drug use, and panic attacks.

The fastest growing population of adults with HIV infection are women, many of whom have children and are single heads of households. One or more of their children may also be infected and, therefore, difficult to place when the mother is hospitalized. Many of these families also face the challenge of maternal injecting drug use.

As a mother's condition progresses to AIDS, she and her family may benefit from family therapy to help cope with a range of issues, including the emotional upheaval inherent in a fatal condition, difficulties adjusting to family life as the mother's parenting abilities decline, and the children's acceptance of new caretakers. Neuropsychological assessment may be needed to determine the mother's ability to continue parental responsibilities, and psychological evaluation may be needed to determine custody or placement. (See Chapter 15, "Women and HIV.")

Many infected persons could benefit from case management services given the array of services and support needed. Persons with AIDS will often need help in sorting through the maze of state and federal entitlement programs.

Referrals to AIDS clinics, the public health department, home healthcare agencies, social services, volunteer agencies, and even vocational services may be appropriate. In addition, a client may need help in finding employment, housing, legal assistance, transportation, financial assistance, child care services, and other resources. Recreational and occupational therapy are also of benefit for many clients.

As the infection progresses to AIDS, people will be confronted with the added burdens of uncertainty, pain, weakness, disfigurement, multiple losses, dementia, and eventually, death. The person faces the loss of key roles in his or her life, changes in appearance, decline of bodily functions, separation from family or friends, and feelings of anxiety, guilt, anger, and helplessness. Social stigma with resulting alienation may compound these problems. As the illness progresses and hospitalizations become more frequent, thoughts of suicide may occur. Crisis intervention and supportive counseling are essential services for this population of clients. Psychotropic medications may also be of value during the course of the illness. (See Chapter 13, "Suicide Assessment and Intervention with Persons Infected with HIV.")

People with cognitive impairment may need day treatment to maintain functioning and to support the primary caregiver by providing a period of respite from the demands of twenty-four-hour care. Specialized hospice care is sometimes necessary in the later stages of the disease. (See Chapter 9, "Neuropsychological Functioning in HIV Disease.")

Preparation for death should begin while the individual still has the necessary cognitive capacity and emotional strength to make reasonable decisions. However, death and dying therapy should not begin so early that efforts to foster hope and optimism are compromised. Persons with AIDS, however, do need to put their affairs in order and make final plans. The course of the illness is progressive, unpredictable, and probably fatal.

As a way of enhancing autonomy at a time when other aspects of life seem out of control, persons with AIDS can be encouraged to prepare a will and a living will and to plan for their funeral and memorial service. They need to have someone available with whom they can discuss their fears and feelings about death and dying. Mental health professionals can assist them as they move through the stages of coping with their own death. (See Chapter 14, "Preparing for Death.") Clinicians may also facilitate reconciliation with alienated family members and help mediate conflicts between families and current friends and lovers.

Staff Knowledge and Attitudes

It is critical that community mental health workers be at ease in discussing all aspects of HIV and AIDS. Irrational fears, prejudice, and stress can lead to burnout and reduce the quality of services provided. Health and mental health workers help to set the tone and should be examples for others in the community for appropriate attitudes and practices regarding HIV.

Nevertheless, mental health workers have reported reluctance to work with HIV-infected individuals, citing fear of contagion and discomfort in working with the terminally ill, injecting drug users, and homosexuals. Despite the large body of literature assuring minimal risk of virus transmission during healthcare procedures, some professionals remain skeptical. Even when the worker is confident of the safety of the job, family and friends may pressure the provider to make professional changes that avoid perceived risk.

Professionals must often confront their own values and prejudices when treating individuals who use drugs or engage in homosexual behavior. Some may have a tendency to blame patients when they have become infected as a result of their own behavior. This may make it difficult to respond with the necessary compassion.

Other characteristics of persons with AIDS may also challenge healthcare workers' abilities to provide quality care. Since persons with AIDS are often young, it may be easy for young healthcare professionals to overidentify with them. Even when maintaining appropriate professional distance, the death of clients may provoke a sense of personal loss in caregivers. The unpredictable course of the disease may lead to feelings of uncertainty for clinicians just as it does for infected individuals and family members. The ever-increasing numbers of clients who have HIV may also lead to a sense of being overwhelmed.

Conclusion

This chapter reviews HIV-related mental health needs and the range of clientele who require services. The development of appropriate and specialized services should be a high priority for CMHCs. The following table lists twenty-seven HIV-related community mental health services associated with each level of the HIV mental health spectrum. These services should be available in all communities.

Spectrum Level Involved

General Community	Healthcare Workers	Significant Others	At Risk	HIV, Asymptomatic	Early Manifestations	Significant Symptoms, Dying	Mental Health Service
	X	X	X	X	X	X	Crisis Intervention
	X	X	X	X	X	X	Psychological Evaluation
	X			X	X	X	Suicide Risk Assessment
	X	X	X	X	X	X	Individual Psychotherapy
	X	X	X	X	X	X	Couples Psychotherapy
	X	X	X	X	X	X	Family Psychotherapy
	X			X	X	X	Child Therapy
	X	X	X	X	X	X	Group Psychotherapy
	X	X	X	X	X	X	Support Groups
			X	X	X		Substance Abuse Treatment
			X	X	X		Client Education
	X	X	X	X	X	X	Stress Management Training
					X	X	Neuropsychological Assessment
						X	Memory Enhancement Training
	X	X					Caregiver Training
		X			X	X	Recreational Therapy
		X			X		Occupational Therapy
		X			X	X	Psychotropic Medication
		X	X		X	X	Case Management
					X	X	Day Treatment
		X				X	Respite Care
						X	Hospice
		X				X	Death and Dying Therapy
		X				X	Bereavement Counseling
X	X	X	X	X	X	X	Risk Reduction Education
X	X	X	X				Community Education
X	X	X	X	X	X	X	Consultation with Health Professionals

TABLE 1.1 HIV-Related Community Mental Health Services Associated with Each Level of the HIV Mental Health Spectrum
Adapted from Knox, M.D., Davis, M., & Friedrich, M.A. (1994).

Review Questions

1. Why are there more people in need of HIV-related mental health care than there are people requiring HIV-related medical care?

2. Name at least five groups of people who may need HIV-related community mental health services.

3. What are some common psychological stressors faced by HIV-spectrum clients?

4. Name three HIV-related community mental health services that could be made available to healthcare providers.

5. List at least six HIV-related community mental health services that may be needed by persons with HIV disease.

References and Suggested Readings

Berman, J.D. (1994). Can community mental health centers meet the challenge of HIV? A Response to Knox, Davis, & Friedrich. *Community Mental Health Journal, 30,* 91–94.

Dow, M., & Knox, M.D. (1991). Mental health and substance abuse staff: HIV/AIDS knowledge and attitudes. *AIDS Care, 3,* 75–87.

Gaies, J., & Knox, M.D. (1991). The therapist and the dying client. *Focus: A Guide to AIDS Research and Counseling, 6*(6), 1–2.

Goldfinger, S. (1990). *Psychiatric Aspects of AIDS and HIV Infection: New Directions for Mental Health Services.* San Francisco: Jossey-Bass.

Kalichman, S.C., Kelly, J.A., Johnson, J.R., & Bulto, M. (1994). Factors associated with risk for HIV infection among chronic mentally ill adults. *American Journal of Psychiatry, 151*(2), 221–227.

Kelly, J.A., Murphy, D.A., Sikkema, K.J., Somlai, A.M., Mulry, G., Fernandez, M.I., Miller, J.G., & Stevenson, L.Y. (1995). Predictors of high and low levels of HIV risk behavior among adults with chronic mental illness. *Psychiatric Services, 46*(8), 813–818.

Kelly, J.A., Sikkema, K.J., Winnet, R.A., Solomon, L.J., Roffman, R.A., Heckman, T.G., Stevenson, L.Y., Perry, M.J., Norman, A.D., & Desirato, L.J. (1995). Factors predicting continued high-risk behavior among gay men in small cities: Psychological, behavioral, and demographic characteristics related to unsafe sex. *Journal of Consulting and Clinical Psychology, 63,* 101–107.

Knox, M.D. (1989). Community mental health's role in the AIDS crisis. *Community Mental Health Journal, 25*(3), 185–196.

Knox, M.D., Boaz, T., Friedrich, M.A., & Dow, M. (1994). HIV risk factors for persons with serious mental illness. *Community Mental Health Journal, 30*(6), 551–563.

Knox, M.D., & Clark, C. (1991). Early HIV detection: A community mental health role. *Journal of Mental Health Administration, 18*(1), 21–26.

Knox, M.D., Davis, M., & Friedrich, M.A. (1994). The HIV mental health spectrum. *Community Mental Health Journal, 30*(1), 75–89.

Knox, M.D., Dow, M., & Cotton, D. (1989). Mental health care providers: The need for AIDS education. *AIDS Education and Prevention, 1,* 285–290.

Knox, M.D., Friedrich, M.A., Gaies, J.S., & Achenbach, K. (1994). Training HIV specialists for community mental health. *Community Mental Health Journal, 30*(4), 405–413.

Knox, L.P., & Knox, M.D. (1995). *Last Wishes: A Handbook to Guide Your Survivors.* Berkeley, CA: Ulysses Press.

Knox, M.D., & Gaies, J. (1990). The HIV clinical tutorial for community mental health professionals. *Community Mental Health Journal, 26*(6), 559–566.

Miller, T., Booraem, C., Flowers, J., & Iverson, A. (1990). Changes in knowledge, attitudes, and behavior as a result of a community-based AIDS prevention program. *AIDS—Education and Prevention, 2,* 12–23.

Morin, S.F. (1988). AIDS: The challenge to psychology. *American Psychologist, 43,* 838–842.

Pollack, D.A. (1994). Comments on training HIV specialists for community mental health. *Community Mental Health Journal, 30,* 415–417.

Sacks, M., Dermatis, H., Looser-Ott, S., Burton, W., & Perry, S. (1992). Undetected HIV infection among acutely ill psychiatric inpatients. *American Journal of Psychiatry, 149,* 544–545.

Chapter 2

The Etiology and Epidemiology of HIV Disease

Kathleen Miner, Ph.D., M.P.H.

Overview

This chapter reviews the origins of HIV disease and the early efforts to understand the opportunistic infections that were eventually called AIDS. The development of the Centers for Disease Control and Prevention (CDC) classification of cases is discussed. Transmission characteristics, the process of HIV testing, and the development of chemotherapy are also included.

The epidemiology of HIV, in the United States and internationally, and the activities of the CDC and the World Health Organization (WHO) are discussed. Common epidemiologic terms are defined and are included at the end of the chapter.

Learning Objectives

1. To recount the origins of the HIV epidemic in the United States.

2. To describe how HIV reaches the immune system.

3. To explain how HIV is transmitted.

4. To understand the differences between the HIV epidemic in the United States and that in the rest of the world.

5. To define at least one epidemiological term.

Outline

   I. The Public Health Approach

  II. Etiology: The Natural History of HIV Disease
- A. History of HIV/AIDS
  1. First cases
  2. Identification and pathogenesis of the human retrovirus
  3. Development of serological testing
  4. Testing of the United States blood supply
  5. Classification of the disease process
- B. Transmission characteristics
  1. Sexual
  2. Needle use
  3. Blood transfusion
  4. Perinatal
  5. Casual contact
  6. Cofactors
     a. Sexually Transmitted Diseases
     b. Substance use

 III. Epidemiology of AIDS
- A. AIDS in the United States
- B. Role of the Centers for Disease Control and Prevention
- C. The international picture

 IV. Definition of Epidemiological Terms
- A. Incidence
- B. Incidence rate
- C. Prevalence
- D. Prevalence rate
- E. Population-based approach
- F. Relative risk
- G. Surveillance
- H. Potential years of life lost

The Public Health Approach

The public health approach to the study of any disease is to investigate the effect of the disease on a population. Because public health is a population-based science, it uses procedures that are quantitative and extend beyond those used in the clinical delivery of healthcare. The analytic techniques used in public health describe the distribution of a particular disease in a group of people and characterize the factors that influence this distribution. These methods are collectively called epidemiology and the investigators that use them are called epidemiologists.

The basis of any epidemiologic investigation is the occurrence of a disease in persons, places, and time. The outcome of the investigation is the identification of the characteristics of who contracted the disease and who did not, whether or not one geographic area had a higher incidence of the disease than others, and whether or not there had been a shift in the occurrence of the disease over time. The science of epidemiology provides the bases upon which the origin, cause, and patterns of diseases are ascertained. This chapter presents an overview of the results of epidemiologic investigations of HIV/AIDS.

Etiology: The Natural History of the Disease

History of HIV/AIDS

Although the term *AIDS* had not yet been coined, the first case of "AIDS" was reported by the CDC in 1981. Soon afterward, physicians in New York and San Francisco began identifying a number of homosexual men with a cancer called Kaposi's sarcoma. The occurrence of this form of cancer in young men was highly unusual. Kaposi's sarcoma is typically found in older adults, people of Mediterranean ancestry, and individuals with compromised immune systems. In addition to the rare form of cancer, homosexual men were presenting with other unusual conditions associated with diminished immune systems, such as a pneumonia caused by *Pneumocystis carinii* and fungus infections of the throat called esophageal candidiasis. Because the early cases were identified in gay men, the disease was initially called gay-related immune disease (GRID). As more cases were identified in populations other than gay men, the term GRID was changed to AIDS (acquired immune deficiency syndrome). It is a peculiarity of the HIV epidemic that the early cases in the United States were identified in the homosexual community. In most of the world, the majority of cases have been among heterosexuals.

During the early 1980s, most of the cases in the United States (nearly 80%) were from six large cities in five states: New York, San Francisco, Los Angeles, Newark, Miami, and Houston. By the end of the 1980s, cases of AIDS had been reported from every state, United States territory, and large city. The CDC classifies the reported AIDS cases by the cities and the states with populations of more than 500,000 in which the individuals were first identified with the disease. Over time these data monitor the spread of the disease through the country. By the middle of 1996, more than fifty metropolitan areas reported a cumulative incidence of over 1,000 cases.

In 1996, by the end of December, 573,800 persons aged 13 years or older with AIDS had been reported to the CDC by United States state and territorial health departments. Male adult and adolescent cases total 488,300, with the remainder (85,500) occurring in women over the age of 13 at the time of diagnosis. The rate of AIDS case identification in the United States is accelerating; 10 percent were identified in the period 1981–87, 41 percent in 1988–92, and 49 percent from 1993 through 1995. During 1996, the estimated number of AIDS deaths was 13 percent lower than the previous year. Much of this decrease is directly attributable to improved chemotherapy coupled with improved nutritional and environmental conditions. Yet despite these improvements, 62 percent of the people who have been diagnosed with AIDS have died. This means that approximately 100 people die each day from AIDS-related causes, translating into one United States AIDS death every 15 minutes.

Based upon the data collected by state health departments throughout the United States, projections of the number of AIDS cases describe an increasing number of cases in women, children, adolescents, heterosexuals, injecting drug users, and people of color. AIDS has become one of the leading causes of potential years of life lost in young adults and adolescents in the United States.

In addition to being a new disease in humans, HIV/AIDS is a dynamic disease. The data describing the HIV/AIDS epidemic constantly change. HIV/AIDS also has social and political consequences that influence the timeliness of reporting cases to public health agencies. The data included in this chapter reflect the latest national and international aggregates in HIV/AIDS reporting. These data age rapidly. To obtain the most current HIV/AIDS data, a number of sources are useful. The CDC publishes a biannual document, *HIV/AIDS Surveillance Report,* that outlines the epidemiology of HIV/AIDS in the United States. The CDC also publishes the *Morbidity and Mortality Weekly Report (MMWR)* that describes new disease trends including information related to HIV/AIDS. Other sources of HIV/AIDS information include the CDC articles and reports posted on the World Wide Web, *http://www.cdc.gov* and the CDC National AIDS Clearinghouse NAC-FAX information system *1-800-458-5231.* Confidential information, referrals, and educational materials on AIDS are available from the CDC National AIDS Hotline *1-800-342-2437, 1-800-344-7432* (Spanish), and *1-800-243-7889* (TTY). Data

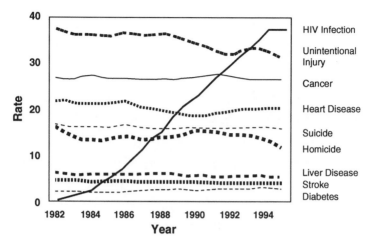

* Per 100,000 population.
** Based on underlying cause of death reported on death certificates, using final data for 1982-1994 and preliminary data for 1995.

Reprinted from Centers for Disease Control and Prevention (1997).

FIGURE 2.1 Death rates (per 100,000 population) for leading causes of death among persons age 25–44 years, by year, United States, 1982–95.

that specify the epidemiology of HIV/AIDS at a state or local level are available from individual state health departments.

Identification and Pathogenesis of the Human Retrovirus

Scientific research teams in France and the United States first isolated the human immunodeficiency virus (HIV) in 1983. Figure 2.2 shows the structure of the human immunodeficiency virus.

All viruses have an outer envelope, called a protein coat, and a core containing one type of nucleic acid, either DNA or RNA. HIV has its genetic material in the form of RNA and is a retrovirus because this must be transcribed into DNA before it becomes functional. Retroviruses have a very rapid rate of genetic mutation, which makes developing a vaccine against them more difficult than developing a vaccine against viruses with DNA in their cores.

HIV selectively infects certain cells in the human body. The primary sites of HIV infection are the white blood cells called T-helper (CD4) lymphocytes and the macrophages. Figure 2.3 shows a virus attacking a CD4 lymphocyte. HIV infection results in the selective destruction of these lymphocytes, which are essential for normal immune function. The illustration also shows the virus replicating in the lymphocyte, destroying the cell, and being released to potentially infect other lymphocytes.

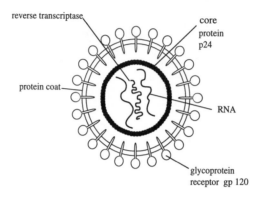

FIGURE 2.2 Structure of the human immunodeficiency virus.

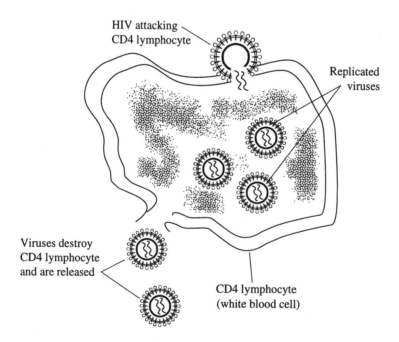

FIGURE 2.3 HIV attacking cell and reproducing new virus.

The clinical disease symptoms associated with HIV infection are the direct result of the destruction of the CD4 lymphocytes. Without these lymphocytes, individuals can no longer mount an effective defense against infectious microorganisms, and they may become ill from diseases that do not usually occur in humans. Many of the diseases associated with AIDS are called opportunistic infections because they are caused by microorganisms that are present, but do not usually cause disease. When an immune system is diminished, the microorganisms that cause *Pneumocystis carinii* pneumonia, candidiasis, toxoplasmosis, and other AIDS-related infections can become pathogenic.

With HIV infection, not all CD4 lymphocytes are destroyed at once. The human body continues to make more CD4 cells that continue to recognize HIV as a pathogen and respond by making specific antibodies against it. As the numbers of virus particles increase, the body gradually loses its ability to generate sufficient numbers of lymphocytes. The average time from first infection with HIV to the inability of the body to keep an adequate supply of lymphocytes is currently about ten years.

HIV is also capable of directly infecting other cells besides the lymphocytes. Brain cells and peripheral nerve cells are common sites of infection by both HIV and opportunistic microorganisms.

Development of Serological Testing

Advances in characterizing the structure of the human immunodeficiency virus permitted researchers to develop techniques for testing blood for the presence of HIV infection. These tests identify the antibody that the lymphocytes make in response to the presence of HIV. The first commercial tests for HIV became available in 1985. They were used to screen the donated blood supply and to determine the presence of HIV infection in individuals.

The two most widely used tests are the enzyme-linked immunosorbent assay (ELISA) and the Western blot. Both tests use blood drawn from the individual. The ELISA is less specific than the Western blot, which means that it has a greater chance of falsely identifying a person as HIV-infected. However, because the ELISA is cheaper, faster, and easier to do, it is used as a first screen of the blood. HIV testing protocols call for a second ELISA if the first ELISA produces a positive reading. If the second ELISA is also positive, the blood is tested using the more specific Western blot to confirm that the blood has evidence of the HIV antibody. Therefore, individuals are considered to be infected with HIV only after their blood has produced two positive ELISAs and one positive Western blot.

It is important to note that a negative result from the ELISA does not mean that the individual is free from HIV. Because the ELISA tests for the presence or absence of the antibody to HIV, there is a chance of a false-negative result if the level of antibody in the blood is very low. If individuals are newly infected with HIV, their lymphocytes may not have produced sufficient amounts of antibody to be detected. Yet, they are still capable of transmitting the virus to others. Generally, it takes from six weeks to several months for antibodies to be produced at levels that can be reliably measured.

During the middle 1990s, there have been other important advances in testing for the presence of HIV. New methods include directly testing for the presence of the virus and its components in blood or tissue, testing for the viral metabolites in the urine, and testing for HIV antibodies in saliva. As these testing procedures become more accurate and less expensive, they will give rise to quicker identification of infection. There is a role for community mental health clinicians in providing post-test counseling to persons using these methods, especially those using home testing kits.

Testing of the United States Blood Supply

Since 1985, there has been universal testing of donated blood in the United States. The standard procedures for collecting and processing blood include self-disclosure of HIV risk factors by donors and testing for HIV using the ELISA or similar tests. A minimal risk of transmitting HIV through blood transfusions remains (2/1,000,000 units). This risk is so low that the United States blood supply is considered safe.

Classification of the Disease Process

The classification of HIV disease has gone through a series of changes as we learned more about the disease process. The earliest system classified the illness according to the type and degree of symptoms present in individuals. As more was learned about the disease, the CDC revised the case definition of AIDS in 1986 and again in 1987.

Summary of the 1987 CDC HIV Classification System

- ■ *Group I.* Acute Infection
- ■ *Group II.* Asymptomatic Infection
- ■ *Group III.* Persistent Generalized Lymphadenopathy
- ■ *Group IV.* Other Diseases:
  Subgroup A. Constitutional Disease
  Subgroup B. Neurologic Disease
  Subgroup C. Secondary Infectious Diseases

Subgroup D. Secondary Cancers

Subgroup E. Other Conditions

The above summary indicates that, through the use of clinical symptoms and laboratory findings, the revised system views AIDS as a chronological progression of HIV infection.

This classification system attempts to place people into four "mutually exclusive groups" of disease status. Group I is the initial stage of infection. Symptoms related to this stage are similar to those of mononucleosis. Group II is the long period between infection and onset of symptoms. Group III people have enlarged lymph nodes. Group IV includes people with any of the diseases in the five subgroups. It is important to note that these diseases can also occur in individuals who are not infected with HIV, but have other reasons for immune suppression or other health problems.

Subgroup A includes persistent fever and involuntary weight loss greater than 10% of total body weight. Subgroup B includes dementia, myelopathy, and peripheral neuropathy. Subgroup C includes symptomatic and invasive diseases such as *Pneumocystis* pneumonia, candidiasis, histoplasmosis, oral hairy leukoplakia, herpes zoster, and others. Subgroup D includes those cancers, associated with diminished immune functioning, such as Kaposi's sarcoma, non-Hodgkin's lymphoma, or primary lymphoma of the brain. Subgroup E includes those diseases or clinical findings not identified in the other subgroups, that are indicative of diminished immune functioning, or that are complications of HIV infection, such as chronic lymphoid interstitial pneumonia.

In 1993, the CDC revised the classification system for HIV disease which provides uniform criteria for staging the progress of the disease in males, females, and adolescents. The revision incorporates serologic counting of the numbers of CD4 lymphocytes. When the CD4 count decreases to 200 or fewer cells per cubic millimeter of blood, the individual is considered to have AIDS.

Transmission Characteristics

HIV has been isolated from a variety of body fluids, including blood, semen, vaginal secretions, breast milk, urine, tears, and saliva. Clearly, any body substance that contains lymphocytes has the possibility of transmitting the virus. Although the virus has been found in all of the body fluids listed above, the amount of virus is very small in tears, urine, and saliva, and the prospect of transmission through casual contact with these fluids is unlikely. Activities that result in contact with blood, blood products, semen, vaginal secretions, and breast milk do carry a significant risk of infection with the virus.

Sexual

Transmission of the virus through sexual contact occurs in both homosexual and heterosexual activities. Any differences between the risk of transmission by penile/vaginal and penile/anal contact are too small to accurately measure. While evidence does suggest that the sexual partner who is the recipient of the semen has a greater risk of becoming infected than the donating partner, transmission in both directions has been unequivocally demonstrated. This evidence appears to hold true for both homosexual and heterosexual contacts. Additional data suggest that individuals who have genital lesions from syphilis or other sexually transmitted diseases (STDs) are at a much increased risk for both transmitting and becoming infected by HIV. Sexual activities that result in the rupture of tissue or the presence of blood may also increase the risk of HIV transmission.

Needle Use

Transmission of the virus through injecting drug use is very efficient and effective. The sharing of blood-contaminated needles, syringes, and drug paraphernalia between an infected person and a noninfected person amounts to a direct inoculation of HIV. The risk of infection is related to the amount of virus that is transmitted. This is the impetus for bleach distribution for cleaning drug paraphernalia and for needle exchange programs.

Blood Transfusion

A blood transfusion containing HIV provides a large inoculation of virus. People receiving infected transfusions almost certainly develop HIV infection. This was the impetus to begin testing the United States blood supply for evidence of HIV as soon as a test was available. Because of their need to stop excessive bleeding, persons with hemophilia must undergo frequent transfusions with concentrated blood products. Before the universal testing of the blood supply, most persons with hemophilia were transfused with multiple doses of infected blood. As a result, many of them developed AIDS. Since the testing of the blood supply for HIV was initiated, this is no longer a significant problem.

Perinatal

Transmission from infected mothers to their children can occur during fetal development, during delivery, and during breast-feeding. Multiple studies indicate that the risk of transmission of the virus from a woman to her fetus is between 15 and 30 percent. The use of anti-HIV drugs during pregnancy appears to significantly reduce the risk of transmission of the virus from an infected woman to the fetus. The precise risk of transmission during delivery and breast-feeding is not known. Because of the presence of large numbers of lymphocytes in breast milk, it is recommended that mothers who are infected not breast-feed their infants.

Casual Contact

There is no evidence that HIV is transmitted through casual contact, food, water, insect bites, or breathing the same air. Hugging, kissing, bathing, and/or living with an HIV-infected person does not result in transmission.

In 1997, the CDC confirmed a case of HIV transmission through deep kissing and the presence of blood in the saliva. It appears that blood was the source of the transmission and not the saliva.

Cofactors

Transmission cofactors are those conditions that do not directly result in HIV infection, but that do increase the likelihood that the virus will be transmitted. STDs such as syphilis and chlamydia are a cofactor. Many of these cause genital sores or ulcers that clearly increase transmission. Substance use is another cofactor. In addition to needle sharing with injecting drug use, many noninjectable drugs, such as alcohol, are considered cofactors for HIV transmission. These substances impair judgment and increase impulsiveness, which increases the probability of engaging in unprotected sexual behaviors that transmit HIV. Moreover, to obtain drugs, many men and women participate in "sex for drugs" exchanges that place them at risk for contacting STDs, including HIV infection.

Epidemiology of AIDS

AIDS in the United States

The total number of United States AIDS cases has exceeded one-half million. Among persons 25–44 years of age, AIDS is now the leading cause of death in men and the third leading cause of death in women. The following chart shows cumulative AIDS cases, by age at the time of diagnosis through December 1996. More than 60 percent of persons with AIDS were diagnosed between the ages of 20 and 39. Twenty-five percent of the cases were in their 40s at the time of diagnosis.

The total number of new AIDS cases reported for 1996 alone was 69,151, which represents an incidence rate of 25.6/100,000 population. As has been true throughout the duration of the AIDS epidemic, more than half of these cases occurred in homosexual/bisexual men.

However, the proportion of AIDS cases attributable to homosexual/bisexual transmission had decreased from 55 percent in early 1994 to 42 percent of new cases by the beginning of 1996. During this same time, there has been a proportional increase of AIDS cases among women and among heterosexual men who were injecting drug users. The trend toward increased heterosexual transmission is expected to continue throughout the rest of the 1990s.

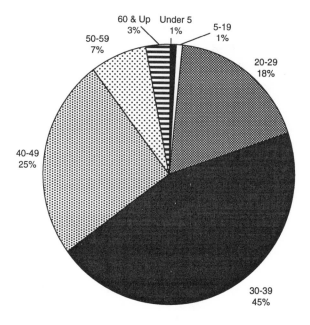

FIGURE 2.4 Cumulative U.S. AIDS cases by age at time of diagnosis, through December 1996.

In addition to the shifts in transmission category, the ethnic composition of the epidemic is changing as well. Although African Americans account for 12 percent of the United States population and Hispanics account for 9 percent, they represent 35 percent and 18 percent, respectively, of the AIDS cases.

AIDS cases in women, children, and adolescents are also increasing. Although cases of AIDS among women were nearly nonexistent in the early years of the epidemic, by December 1996 women accounted for 15 percent of cumulative cases. Children and adolescents accounted for 1 percent of cumulative United States AIDS cases.

There also have been dramatic shifts in the regional patterns of AIDS cases. The South has had significant increases in reported cases among homosexual/bisexual men, women, and heterosexuals. No longer are rural communities exempt. By December 1996, nonmetropolitan areas reported 6 percent of all AIDS cases.

Role of the Centers for Disease Control and Prevention

The Centers for Disease Control and Prevention is the agency of the United States federal government responsible for monitoring the AIDS epidemic. It publishes monthly and quarterly updates on the reported incidence, incidence rates,

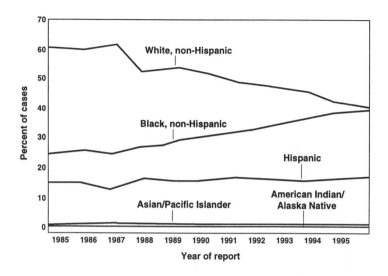

FIGURE 2.5 Percentage of U.S. AIDS cases by race/ethnicity/and year of report, 1985–95. Reprinted from Centers for Disease Control and Prevention (1995)

prevalence, and prevalence rates for AIDS cases in the United States. From 1981 through December 1996, the total number of persons with AIDS reported to the CDC was 581,429. The CDC investigates suspected transmissions of HIV to determine whether or not new transmission routes exist. The CDC is studying possible HIV transmissions associated with medical and dental treatments provided by infected healthcare workers to their patients, as well as from patients to providers. Although the results of these studies remain inconclusive, there is little evidence to suggest that this is a significant method of viral transmission.

The number of AIDS cases is not a true measure of the scope of the epidemic. The real indicator of the severity of the problem is the number of persons who are infected with the virus. Because of confidential and anonymous HIV reporting protocols, it is impossible to state conclusively how many people are infected with HIV. Through the use of projections and special studies, the CDC estimates that the number of United States citizens infected with HIV, but not yet diagnosed with AIDS, could be as high as 1,000,000.

Future trends in HIV/AIDS prevalence will be influenced by the availability and effectiveness of interventions that will prevent new infections, promote early diagnosis, and facilitate advances in the medical management of the disease. The ability to design, implement, and evaluate these interventions will require consistent long-term funding, access to accurate data, and availability of trained personnel who can use these data in making programmatic decisions.

The International Picture

The World Health Organization (WHO) is the international agency responsible for monitoring the global status of HIV/AIDS. WHO is part of the United Nations and has its headquarters in Geneva, Switzerland. WHO estimates that 18.5 million adults and 1.5 million children are infected with HIV. Although the WHO reporting system has identified 1,291,810 cases of AIDS, delays in accounting coupled with the economic and political obstacles of identifying infected persons make underreporting a severe problem. WHO estimates that as many as 4.5 million people have developed full-blown AIDS. HIV is present in all countries of the world, and cases of AIDS have been reported from every country as well. Despite efforts to limit its spread, the HIV epidemic continues to expand rapidly. Every day there are approximately 6,000 new infections. Additionally, as the disease expands its range, a greater proportion of new cases will be among women and children.

The global picture of AIDS differs from the United States epidemic in a number of ways. The most striking indication of these differences is the mode of transmission. In the United States, homosexual transmission is the most frequent means, however; worldwide it accounts for less than 15 percent of AIDS cases. Although increasing in the United States, heterosexual transmission accounts for about 10 percent of the United States AIDS cases, but internationally accounts for more than 70 percent.

In much of the developing world, the financial resources available for AIDS treatment are miniscule. In countries where the annual per capita healthcare expenditure is less than $2.00 in United States currency, it is impossible to provide expensive treatment to infected persons. Moreover, the high incidence of AIDS in both men and women increases the likelihood that children will be born infected or will be orphaned by the death of their infected parents. By the year 2000, WHO predicts that between 5 and 10 million children will have lost both parents because of AIDS.

It is evident that knowledge of HIV/AIDS is not sufficient enough to change human behavior. For many people, the social, environmental, and economic factors are powerful pressures to engage in behaviors that risk the transmission of the virus. The three strategies that hold promise for the global control of the AIDS pandemic are:

1. Support the availability of condoms and demystify their use.

2. Assist communities to implement local models of healthcare delivery.

3. Encourage the adoption of safer sex practices and increase the economic and social power of women and youth.

Definition of Epidemiological Terms

The following epidemiologic terms are used by public health professions to describe the status of a particular disease. These definitions are adapted from those cited in *A Dictionary of Epidemiology.*

Incidence

The incidence of a disease represents the number of new cases of a disease in a defined population within a specified period of time. With AIDS, the defined populations include the total population of a geographic area (country, state, county, city) and the major gender, behavioral, ethnic, and age segments of a population, such as women, homosexuals, injecting drug users, and children. The usual time period associated with incidence is one year, although shorter (months) or longer (5–10 years) periods of time may be used, depending upon the nature of the disease. For example, the number of people aged 13 or older reported with AIDS in 1996 was 68,473 and the total number of United States AIDS cases reported from April 1981 through December 1996 was 581,429.

Incidence Rate

Incidence rate refers to the rate at which new cases of disease occur in a population during a specified time period. The rate implies a mathematical calculation. In this case, the numerator is the number of new cases, and the denominator is the number of individuals in the population who are at risk or who could get the disease. Often the population used in the denominator is standardized to a number that is a multiple of 10. This allows for a common comparison across populations. An illustration of this would be as follows: During 1995, the incidence rate of AIDS-related opportunistic infections was 99 per 100,000 for non-Hispanic blacks, 50 per 100,000 Hispanics, and 15 per 100,000 non-Hispanic whites. Sometimes it is helpful to determine the incidence rate associated with a particular mode of exposure. For example, if 1,000 people experience needlesticks with contaminated needles, 4 of these people would be expected to develop HIV infection. This is because the incidence rate for needlestick injuries is 1 in 250. With HIV, the incidence rate is useful in determining the likelihood that someone will become infected as the result of a particular exposure to HIV.

Prevalence

Prevalence of a disease represents the total number of cases (both new and previously diagnosed) of a disease at a designated time. With AIDS, prevalence can be used to describe the numbers of persons who have been diagnosed with the disease and who are still alive and reside in a particular community. This is useful in determining the number of individuals who will be needing services and other forms of support. Prevalence is calculated by counting the number of new cases and adding these cases to the number of previously diagnosed cases and subtracting the number of individuals who have died. For example, as of June 1996 the prevalence of AIDS was 223,000 United States residents aged 13 years and older.

Prevalence Rate

Just as with an incidence rate, a prevalence rate is a mathematical calculation of dividing a numerator by a denominator in a given time period. Prevalence rate is the total number of cases of the condition or disease in the numerator, divided by the population at risk of having the condition or disease in the denominator. Often the denominator is the population of the entire community of interest. For example, the prevalence rate of AIDS in the United States per 100,000 residents for 1994–95 was 29.1.

Population-Based Approach

Population-based surveillance is the basic approach used in epidemiology that selects the population of a geographical region or social boundary as the sampling frame for studies. This same population is used as the denominator in analyses. This is different from many medical studies that look only at patients and no one else in the community. With HIV disease, the use of a population-based approach provides insight into the number of people needing services in a given community.

Relative Risk

Often referred to as a "risk ratio" or "odds ratio," the relative risk is the risk of disease or death in an exposed population as compared with the risk of death or disease in the unexposed population. With HIV infection, relative risk is frequently used to describe the hazard associated with certain behavior. Examples are the relative risk of not using zidovudine (AZT) versus using AZT or the risk of transmitting the virus while not using a condom as opposed to the risk of transmission using a condom. For example, during the clinical trials of AZT, 281 HIV-infected persons were divided into treatment and control groups. After several months of therapy, it was determined that there were nineteen deaths in the control group and only one death in the treatment group; thus the relative risk of death was 19:1.

Surveillance

Surveillance is the close and continuous monitoring of a population to identify new cases of a particular disease. With HIV infection, surveillance is useful in determining new patterns of disease. One example might be documenting the shifting pattern of disease within risk categories, such as from homosexual to heterosexual transmission and from white males to other ethnic groups and women.

Potential Years of Life Lost

This is a calculation that attempts to measure the relative impact of disease or other lethal events on society. Those diseases that cause the death of younger members of society result in a higher rating of potential years of life lost. With AIDS, the impact on society is very large because the majority of AIDS-related deaths occur in younger people.

Review Questions

1. In the United States, what groups of people are showing increased rates of AIDS?

2. How does HIV reach the immune system?

3. How is HIV transmitted?

4. Proportionally, are more women in the United States infected with AIDS than in the rest of the world?

References and Suggested Readings

Centers for Disease Control and Prevention. (1997). *Update: Trends in AIDS Incidence, Deaths, and Prevalence — United States, 1996, 46*(8).

Centers for Disease Control and Prevention. (1997). *HIV/AIDS Surveillance Report, 8*(2).

Centers for Disease Control and Prevention. (1995). *HIV/AIDS Surveillance Report, 7*(2).

Centers for Disease Control and Prevention. (1992). 1993 revised classification system for HIV infection and expanded case definition for AIDS among adolescents and adults. *Morbidity and Mortality Weekly Report, 41*(No. RR-17).

Centers for Disease Control. (1987). Revision of the CDC surveillance case definition for acquired immunodeficiency syndrome. *Morbidity and Mortality Weekly Report, 36*(1S).

Centers for Disease Control. (1986). Current trends: Classification system for human T lymphotropic virus type III/lymphadenopathy associated viral infections. *Morbidity and Mortality Weekly Report, 35*, 334–339.

Centers for Disease Control. (1985). *Morbidity and Mortality Weekly Report, 34,* 373–375.

Centers for Disease Control and Prevention. (1997). *Morbidity and Mortality Weekly Report, 46,* 171.

Centers for Disease Control. (1981). Kaposi's sarcoma and *Pneumocystis* pneumonia among homosexual men—New York City and California. *Morbidity and Mortality Weekly Report, 30,* 305–308.

Chiasson, M., Berenson, L., Li, W., Schwartz, S., Mojica, B., & Hamburg, M. (1997). Declining AIDS mortality in New York City. Abstract. In *Program and Abstracts of the IV Conference on Retroviruses and Opportunistic Infections, 1997.*

Last, J.M. (Ed.) (1988). *A Dictionary of Epidemiology* (2nd ed.). New York: Oxford University Press.

National Commission on AIDS. (1991). *America Living with AIDS: Transforming Anger, Fear and Indifference into Action.* Report of the National Commission on Acquired Immune Deficiency Syndrome. Washington, D.C.: National Commission on AIDS.

Valdiserri, R.O., Aultman, T.V., & Curran, J.W. (1995). Community planning: A national strategy to improve HIV prevention programs. *Journal of Community Health, 20,* 87–100.

Chapter 3

HIV and the Law

Joline Miceli-Mullen, J.D.

Overview

This chapter introduces readers to the legal issues that relate to HIV disease/AIDS. Issues of informed consent, medical confidentiality, duty to warn, and employer liability are reviewed. Legal issues and planning for healthcare and terminal illness are also included.

Learning Objectives

1. To identify prohibited practices under the Americans with Disabilities Act.
2. To understand the concepts of informed consent.
3. To identify the legal elements of the duty to warn.
4. To understand tools adult AIDS patients may use for end of life planning.

Outline

I. The Americans with Disabilities Act
   A. Employment

    B. Public accommodation

II. Patient Care Issues

    A. Informed consent

    B. Confidentiality of medical and HIV information

    C. Duty to warn

    D. Providers with HIV disease

III. Death and Advance Planning

    A. Living wills

    B. Healthcare surrogates

    C. Durable powers of attorney

NOTE: There are many federal and state laws addressing issues related to HIV disease. State laws will vary. Therefore, some of the details of this chapter may differ from state to state. Please consult legal counsel.

The Americans with Disabilities Act

The Americans with Disabilities Act of 1990 (ADA), which is comprehensive antidiscrimination legislation for persons with disabilities, was signed into law by President George Bush in 1990. This law contains five titles, the most important being Titles I and III. Title I, which prohibits discrimination in employment, and Title III, which deals with places of public accommodation, became effective July 26, 1992. There are also provisions in the law that address public agencies, public transportation, and telecommunications. This chapter is limited to an overview of Titles I and III.

Employment Issues

Under the ADA, employers may not discriminate against qualified individuals with disabilities because of any disability. A disability is a physical or mental impairment that substantially limits one or more major life activities, having a record of such impairment, or being regarded as having such impairment. The prohibition against disability-based discrimination applies to the job application process, hiring, discharge, advancement, compensation, job training, and other terms, conditions, and privileges of employment. Both direct and adverse impact discrimination are proscribed. Employers may not limit, segregate, classify, or use non-job-related screening measures with job applicants or employees in a way that adversely affects job opportunities because of disability. Likewise, participation in any contract or arrangement and adopting any standards, criteria, or policies that have the effect of discriminating based on disability are prohibited by the ADA.

Disability

- Physical or mental impairment
- Limits one or more major life activities
- Record of impairment
- Regarded as having impairment (stereotypes)

Employers are required to make reasonable accommodation for qualified individuals with disabilities to enable them to perform the essential functions of the job. A qualified individual is an individual with a disability who, with or without reasonable accommodation, is able to perform the essential functions of the job held or desired. Accommodations that would impose an undue hardship on the operation of the employer's business are not considered reasonable. Persons who pose a significant risk to the health or safety of others in the workplace which cannot be eliminated by reasonable accommodation may not be qualified individuals.

HIV disease and AIDS are considered disabilities under the law. Thus, the ADA provides protections from discrimination for those with HIV or AIDS. However, if such individuals pose a significant risk of harm to others, ADA protections may not apply. This has been most apparent in healthcare occupations involving invasive procedures.

The following questions and answers deal with issues of discrimination and are provided to assist the reader in identifying prohibited practices under the ADA:

Question 1: Judy, a registered nurse, had tested positive for HIV, and this test result was in her employment record. Judy applied for a job that did not involve any direct patient care contact. With her consent, the record was given to the prospective employer, who decided not to hire Judy because of the HIV-positive result. Was Judy the subject of unlawful discrimination?

Answer 1: Assuming Judy was qualified for the new job, unlawful discrimination did occur. Judy may be rejected for the job if she is not qualified to perform the essential job functions, but not because of her HIV status.

Question 2: Sally, a registered nurse who assists with open-heart surgery, is asymptomatic HIV-positive. A significant and essential part of her job requires her to participate in invasive procedures. Sally strictly adheres to universal precautions. May Sally be terminated because she is HIV-positive?

Answer 2: If there are other vacant jobs within the facility that do not involve invasive procedures and for which Sally is qualified, a reasonable accommodation might be to reassign Sally so that she would not pose a risk of transmission of the virus to patients. If there are no other vacant jobs, a new position does not have to be created for Sally. If Sally poses a significant risk to the health of her patients by participating in invasive procedures, she may be removed from the job. Thus far, courts have permitted similar dismissals.

Question 3: As Sally's disease progresses, she begins to suffer from mental impairment and motor dysfunction, which cause her to become unable to perform her job properly. She is beginning to make improper sutures. Suturing is an essential function of her job. May Sally be removed from her job?

Answer 3: Suturing is an essential function of her job that she is no longer able to perform. Assuming there are not any reasonable accommodations that can be made to cause Sally to be able to perform this function competently, Sally is not qualified. She is not able to perform an essential function of the job.

Public Accommodation Issues

The ADA law is not limited to regulating employers. Owners, operators, and leasees of places of public accommodation whose operations affect commerce are also prohibited from discriminating on the basis of disability. They may not deny or provide unequal or separate goods, services, benefits, or privileges to individuals on the basis of their disability. Different or separate services may be provided to persons with disabilities when necessary to ensure disabled persons' access to the services. However, persons with disabilities must have the opportunity to participate in either service.

Physician and other healthcare provider offices, as well as hospitals and healthcare facilities, are specifically included in the law as places of public accommodation. The definition also includes retail establishments, lodgings, eateries, theaters, arenas and stadiums, parks, zoos, schools, social centers, gymnasiums, and other public places.

Public Accommodations

- Professional practice offices
- Retail establishments

- Arenas, stadiums, gymnasiums, etc.
- Restaurants and lodgings
- Theaters, museums, and galleries
- Service establishments (salons, cleaners, travel agencies, attorneys' and accountants' offices, etc.)
- Parks, zoos, and recreational places
- Schools, day-care centers, senior centers, etc.

Question 4: Dr. Jones is a board-certified orthopedic physician. Mary, who is HIV-positive, went to Dr. Jones's office for treatment of her dermatological problems associated with HIV infection. Dr. Jones makes it a practice not to treat HIV-positive patients at his office. May he lawfully refuse to treat Mary?

Answer 4: Yes. Although it is unlawful for professional practice offices, as places of public accommodation, to refuse to provide services on the basis of an individual's disability, Dr. Jones may refuse to treat Mary if he is not qualified to treat dermatological problems. However, if Mary had come to Dr. Jones with a hip fracture, a refusal by Dr. Jones to treat Mary's fracture because she is HIV-positive would be unlawful under the ADA.

Patient Care Issues

Informed Consent

In most states, informed consent and pre- and posttest counseling are required, with some exceptions, whenever an HIV test is administered. Informed consent is a process that involves discussing pertinent information with the patient and ensuring that the patient has the right, and understands that he or she has the right, to refuse the proposed treatment or HIV test. Consent must be obtained voluntarily and without undue influence.

While states differ as to the specific information to be provided to patients, it is generally accepted that for consent to be "informed" the patient must be advised of the nature of the procedure, the reasonably foreseeable risks, and the medically acceptable alternatives. For HIV testing, this would entail advising the patient that an HIV test is a blood test, the meaning of both positive and negative results, the risks associated with disclosure of the information, and alternatives such as anonymous testing, where available.

For informed consent to be valid, the patient must have the legal and actual capacity to understand the discussion and give consent. By definition, minors lack this capacity. However, in many states, with respect to HIV testing and certain other situations, minors may give consent. Individuals who are mentally impaired also lack the capacity to consent. Consent may then be obtained from a lawfully authorized representative. Persons who may act as representatives will vary from state to state.

Informed Consent

- Voluntary
- Capacity to understand
- Nature of procedure
- Risks
- Alternatives

In summary, informed consent requires that the consent be voluntarily given by a patient with legal capacity or by a lawfully authorized representative after discussions regarding procedure, risks, and alternatives.

Confidentiality of Medical and HIV Information

Like all medical information, HIV information is confidential. It may not be released except in accordance with law. In many states it is more confidential than usual medical information and is considered "superconfidential." Superconfidential HIV information may be disclosed only as specified by law. Generally, it may be disclosed to those involved with the medical care of the patient who need to know for purposes of treating the patient and to persons who need to know for purposes of doing their jobs. Although state laws differ, superconfidential HIV information usually may not otherwise be disclosed without a court order or the patient's specific authorization. Neither a subpoena or general release will suffice to authorize the release of superconfidential HIV information. All persons who have access to or receive the HIV information of another are held to these requirements of confidentiality. There are other limited situations in each state that allow the sharing of HIV information. These may relate to when a significant exposure occurs, anonymous medical research, and disclosure to significant others. Healthcare providers are not entitled to know a person's HIV status, except as necessary for appropriate diagnosis and treatment of any individual. Under law, healthcare providers may not refuse to provide treatment on the basis of HIV status. Many states forbid healthcare providers and facilities from requiring an HIV test as a condition of treatment, except when the test is necessary to evaluate the appropriateness of specific treatments. Even in this situation, informed consent is required.

Duty to Warn

The duty to warn is a legal obligation created by the landmark case of *Tarasoff v. the Regents of University of California.* Not all states have adopted the duty to warn. Where it has been adopted, it arises when a patient of a licensed health professional threatens to render serious physical harm to an identified individual, and the healthcare provider believes that the patient is capable and intends to carry out the threat. The provider is then obligated to warn the individual or to take reasonable steps to protect him or her from harm. Such steps might include advising law enforcement by providing appropriate information.

Duty to Warn

- Threat of serious physical harm
- By patient
- To identified (or sometimes unidentified) victim
- Likely to occur

Under these circumstances, the healthcare provider may have a legal obligation to violate the patient's confidentiality to protect the nonpatient from harm.

In some states, healthcare providers are allowed to disclose the HIV-positive status of their patients to the sex or needle-sharing partner of the patient if the patient intends to have unprotected sex or share needles without disclosing his or her status to the partner. The provider must first attempt to convince the patient to disclose his or her status to the partner and to refrain from high-risk activity.

Providers with HIV Disease

To date, there are no federal statutes that prohibit infected healthcare providers from continuing in their jobs. In fact, the protections of the ADA would seem to apply to healthcare providers who do not pose a significant risk to the health of others. However, there have been cases where infected providers were discharged from their positions as a result of being HIV-positive. Such cases have primarily involved healthcare providers whose duties include preforming invasive procedures. The courts have taken the position that, when the ultimate harm is death, no risk is acceptable.

The CDC has advised that providers who use universal precautions can continue to perform invasive procedures, but not exposure-prone procedures, without first receiving the patient's informed consent. The CDC did suggest that providers who perform invasive procedures "know their HIVstatus." The CDC guideline is based on the extremely low risk of transmission by providers who use universal precautions. Nonetheless, a trend is in sight under which healthcare providers might be held to a higher degree of responsibility that includes the responsibility to know their HIV status; the responsibility to refrain from performing invasive procedures if they are HIV-positive; and the responsibility to advise their patients of their status.

Death and Advance Planning

Almost every state in the nation recognizes, through statute or case law, some form of advance directive to handle the medical care of persons whose illness renders them incapable of making decisions. Advance directives can take the form of a living will, healthcare surrogate, or durable healthcare power of attorney.

Advance Directives

- Living will
- Healthcare surrogate
- Durable healthcare power of attorney

A living will is a document in which an individual states his or her desires concerning the continuation or discontinuation of medical care should the person become incompetent. It is a statement of wishes concerning medical care, made in advance, and usually concerns life-prolonging procedures. In general, living wills become effective when the patient is suffering from a terminal condition and is no longer capable of making his or her own healthcare decisions.

A healthcare surrogate is a person appointed by an individual to make healthcare decisions on his or her behalf in the event of mental or physical incapacity to communicate knowing and willful healthcare decisions. Once appointed, a healthcare surrogate generally has the authority to make almost all healthcare decisions that the patient could have made if he or she were capable of doing so, including the authority to refuse medical care. A durable healthcare power of attorney is essentially the same as a healthcare surrogate. It is a document by which the patient, while competent, appoints another individual to make healthcare decisions for him or her in the event that he or she becomes incapable of doing so. A durable power of attorney must contain special language indicating it survives the principal's incompetence.

Under principles relating to the right to privacy, some states authorize "proxies" to make healthcare decisions on behalf of patients who are incapable of making healthcare decisions when there has not been a previously executed living will, durable power of attorney for healthcare, or healthcare surrogate. Proxies and surrogates are required to make decisions based on previous oral or written expressions of the patient, if any; what they believe the patient would have wanted; and consideration of the best interests of the patient. There are limitations, in some states, on the surrogate's or proxy's authority. For example, a surrogate generally does not have the authority to consent to an abortion, sterilization, electroshock therapy, or experimental treatments.

Review Questions

1. How does the Americans with Disabilities Act protect persons with HIV disease?

2. Name the elements of informed consent.

3. Under the CDC guidelines of 1991, can healthcare providers continue to perform invasive procedures without the patient knowing the provider's HIV status?

4. What is a healthcare surrogate?

References and Suggested Readings

Americans with Disabilities Act of 1990. Public Laws, 101–336.
Tarasoff v. Regents of University of California, 551 P. 2d 334 (1976).
Behringer v. Medical Center at Princeton, 592 A. 2nd 1251 (N.J. Super. 1991).
Centers for Disease Control (1991). Recommendations for preventing transmission of human immunodeficiency virus and hepatitis B virus to patients during exposure-prone invasive decisions. *Mortality and Morbidity Weekly Report, 40*(No. RR-8), 1–9.
Florida Statutes, Section 381.004.

Chapter 4

Ethics and HIV in Community Mental Health Settings

Frank Chessa, M.A., and
Robert M. Walker, M.D.

Overview

This chapter explains principles of healthcare ethics and how they apply to HIV in community mental health settings. The ethical principles of beneficence, autonomy, justice, and responsibility support the professional commitment to provide mental healthcare. These principles are introduced and used to analyze ethical problems that may arise in community mental health centers (CMHCs). Ethical problems are arranged in four topic areas: attitudes toward HIV; informed consent and testing; confidentiality; and HIV preventive education.

Learning Objectives

1. To identify and define at least two ethical principles that underlie the practice of community mental healthcare.

2. To recognize negative attitudes about HIV that impair appropriate care and to name two strategies that may be used to combat these attitudes.

3. To specify ethical requirements for informed consent for HIV counseling and testing.

4. To specify how to handle HIV test results and HIV/AIDS-related information in a manner that respects confidentiality.

Outline

   I. HIV and Ethics

  II. The Ethics of Treatment
     A. Beneficence
     B. Autonomy
     C. Justice
     D. Responsibility

 III. Negative Attitudes toward HIV

 IV. Ethical Dilemmas in HIV Care
     A. HIV testing and informed consent
       1. General principles guiding the appropriate use of HIV tests
       2. Ethical requirements of informed consent for HIV counseling and testing
     B. Confidentiality
       1. Reasons to maintain confidentiality
       2. Reasons to breach confidentiality
     C. Ethical aspects of HIV prevention and education
       1. Options regarding sex
       2. Options regarding drug use

  V. Conclusion

HIV and Ethics

Ethical questions can present a challenge for CMHC staff. Perhaps you have heard people say, "How can we as a society ensure that all HIV-infected persons will receive compassionate and competent care?" or "Must I care for HIV-infected clients? Can't I refuse? Why should I put myself at risk for getting the infection?" There is seemingly no end to the number of questions: "Isn't my duty to protect myself and my family more important than anything else? Since most people with

HIV have brought it upon themselves, aren't they just getting what they deserve? Why shouldn't we be able to test all clients to make sure they don't have HIV? Why do we have to go through a consent process just to perform a simple blood test for HIV antibodies? Why is HIV status treated with such a high level of confidentiality when other information about medical status is not? Can we reveal a client's HIV status to others who are involved in care?"

The Ethics of Treatment

To answer some of these common questions, it is helpful to review our professional commitment to caring for those with mental health needs and to review the general ethical principles that support that commitment.

Ethical Principles for Community Mental Healthcare

■ Beneficence

■ Autonomy

■ Justice

■ Responsibility

As mental health providers, we are committed to helping those with mental health problems. We offer care on the basis of needs, not on the basis of social acceptance of one's life-style or on the basis of one's particular diagnosis.

The principle that underscores this general orientation is called "beneficence." Beneficence simply means "doing good." As community mental health professionals, it means doing what is in our clients' best interests in terms of their mental health.

A second ethical principle that guides our professional orientation is that of "autonomy" or "respect for persons." When a client comes to us for treatment, we attempt to meet their mental health needs (beneficence) and, at the same time, maintain respect for our client as a fellow human being. We respect their choices, treat them with courtesy and dignity, and avoid any tendency toward depersonalization. We hold, in trust, information the client wishes be kept confidential. We inform and counsel them about HIV testing and respect their decision when they consent to or reject it.

A third principle is "justice" or "fairness." This is the idea that we treat clients with similar mental health needs similarly. We do not discriminate among clients on the basis of our dislike for their life-styles or because of their race or ethnicity. In the case of HIV, the principle of justice means that we do not treat persons with HIV differently from others simply because they have HIV.

Fourth, and last, there is the principle of "responsibility." As mental healthcare providers, we have an obligation to render care in a way that is consistent with the laws of our state and the policies and procedures of our particular health institution. These policies, procedures, and health laws were created to protect the general welfare. In abiding by them, we are fulfilling a general responsibility to society as a whole. Furthermore, when we agreed to train and work as mental healthcare providers, we promised to work within the practice parameters put forth by our profession, our state, and our treatment facility. If we knowingly violate these parameters, we not only fail to live up to our responsibility, but we are breaking that promise.

These four principles reflect the ethical values that healthcare providers endorse as part of their professional commitment. It is possible to imagine circumstances in which two of the principles conflict: for example, when doing what is best for a client (beneficence) runs counter to the client's own wishes (autonomy).

Below, we discuss how some types of conflict related to HIV may be resolved. There is often no easy answer about which principle should "take precedence." Healthcare providers must remember that each principle is important and seek a resolution that minimizes the extent to which any one principle is disregarded. It may be disappointing that the approach guided by these principles may not yield a straightforward answer. However, professional responsibility mandates wise and careful deliberation regarding ethical conflicts. (More information on the use of principles in medical ethics may be found in Beauchamp and Childress (1994) and Gillon (1994).)

Negative Attitudes toward HIV

As we examine some of the issues that arise in HIV care, we will practice applying these four ethical principles. First, negative attitudes impede our ability to live up to the ethical principles that guide mental healthcare. Our ability to render competent and compassionate care to clients can be impaired by negative attitudes toward persons with HIV infection.

These attitudes commonly stem from fear—in particular, the fear of contagion. But negative attitudes also stem from negative judgments about other people. Some persons believe that some people with HIV are "getting what they deserve" because they contracted the virus through perceived immoral, or "bad," behavior. Obviously, if mental healthcare providers allow such attitudes to affect their practice, the care received by HIV-infected persons will be neither competent nor compassionate. Providers who, on these grounds, refuse to care for persons with HIV-infection are not operating under the principle of beneficence. They do not respect the HIV-infected individual as a person, nor do they act under the principle of justice or fairness.

Fear of contagion is largely unjustified in view of the facts concerning modes of HIV transmission. We know how the virus is spread and that it is not spread through the casual contact that characterizes most of our work in CMHCs. In cases where one expects to come into contact with the body fluids (e.g., blood) of an HIV-infected client, one should take universal precautions as recommended by the Centers for Disease Control and Prevention (CDC). Studies have clearly demonstrated the effectiveness of these precautions in preventing spread of the infection from client to provider and vice versa. (See Chapter 6, "HIV Transmission in Healthcare Settings and Infection Control for Healthcare Workers.") In view of these studies, fear of contagion so great that it would keep a mental healthcare provider from rendering appropriate care is unjustified.

Other attitudes are harder to fight with facts. These include negative attitudes regarding the life-styles and behavior of many persons infected with HIV. These attitudes have the potential to impair or impede appropriate treatment. For example, some healthcare providers have refused to be involved in the care of some HIV-infected persons because they believe the homosexual life-style is wrong. Although one may be uncomfortable with different sexual mores, personal attitudes should not get in the way of rendering appropriate care to those who are afflicted with HIV disease.

When negative attitudes impair our ability to deliver appropriate mental healthcare, we may violate the ethical principles of beneficence, autonomy, justice, and responsibility that underlie the entire purpose of mental healthcare. If negative attitudes lead one to refuse involvement in the care of HIV-positive persons, then one abandons the principle of beneficence. And by continuing to care for persons who have similar mental health needs, but who are not HIV-infected, one violates the principle of justice. By refusing needed care to a particular individual, based on life-style or diagnosis, one does not show respect for persons. Indeed, there is a tendency to depersonalize HIV-infected clients, to think of them as "different". Fortunately, studies show that these negative attitudes often decrease with education and with experience in caring for persons with HIV (Gordin et al., 1987; McKinnon, Insall, Gooch, and Cockcroft, 1990; Wertz et al., 1987).

Finally, refusing to care for HIV-infected clients on the basis of their diagnosis, their life-styles, or behavior may be a violation of professional codes of ethics, of state law, or of health facility policy. The practice of excluding HIV-infected persons from appropriate care or of segregating them may be discriminatory and violate the provisions of the Americans with Disabilities Act, a federal law.

Ethical Dilemmas in HIV Care

There are several treatment issues that create ethical dilemmas: HIV testing, client confidentiality, and preventive education.

HIV Testing and Informed Consent

General Principles Guiding the Appropriate Use of HIV Tests
Some people have asserted that everyone should be required to be tested for HIV. They reason that a program of universal testing would be the most effective way to stop the HIV epidemic. However, there are problems with universal testing programs, as the following list shows.

Problems with Universal Testing Programs

- Persons would have to be tested for HIV repeatedly.
- Testing would not identify everyone with HIV.
- Testing everyone for HIV would be expensive.
- It is unclear what, if any, public health benefits would accrue from identifying everyone who is infected.

Because people can become infected with HIV at any time, we would have to test people repeatedly. Even then, HIV testing would never identify everyone with HIV, because a person who has recently been infected will test negative for HIV antibodies for a period of weeks to months. Testing everyone repeatedly would not be cost-effective. Finally, it is not clear what public health benefits would accrue from universal testing, because no reasonable actions could be taken without a gross violation of civil liberties. For example, segregating, quarantining, or imprisoning all infected people would violate the ethical principles discussed in this chapter as well as federal law.

Some may argue that noninfected people should be protected from HIV infection by testing all of the members of a particular group, such as hospital patients, in order to protect healthcare providers from infection. However, the knowledge that a certain patient is infected with HIV would not result in risk reduction for healthcare workers, because no significant risk of transmission exists. Since HIV is not spread through casual contact, aside from accidental needlestick, there is little chance that healthcare workers would become infected from a client. Instead of testing all patients, taking routine precautions is the wise alternative. (See Chapter 6, "HIV Transmission in Healthcare Settings and Infection Control for Healthcare Workers.")

If it is not useful or feasible to test everyone for HIV, then one might try to set out the circumstances in which it is appropriate to test for HIV. Let us apply the ethical principles already introduced.

Beneficence implies that a medical procedure ought to benefit the person for whom the procedure is being done. In other words, HIV testing should be performed primarily because it benefits the client. The principle of beneficence is served if caregivers encourage HIV testing, because being tested for HIV is more likely than ever before to be in the best interest of a patient. Recent advances in antiretroviral therapies have made it possible to dramatically slow the progression of HIV disease (Deeks, Smith, Holodniy, and Kahn, 1997). In addition, encouraging a patient to be tested for HIV carries an implicit promise to be available to assist the patient should the test be positive. (See Chapter 5, "The Clinician's Role in Early Detection of HIV.")

Autonomy implies that people are entitled to make decisions about medical procedures that affect their own physical or mental well-being. We generally recognize this as part of an individual's "freedom" to make choices, an important element of what it is to be a person. Sometimes, such as in an emergency, the principle of autonomy is bypassed to prevent harm to the client, but, in most cases, a person has the right to make decisions regarding his or her own healthcare. Each individual should be able to decide whether or not he or she will undergo testing for HIV.

First and foremost, the client's own feelings about testing should be assessed. Does the client wish to be tested? So that he or she can assess their personal risk, does the client understand how HIV is transmitted? If a healthcare worker feels that there is a good reason to test for HIV, the caregiver should explain these reasons to the client so that an informed choice can be made. Explaining why an HIV test is a good idea and assessing the client's willingness to take the test serve to promote the client's autonomy.

Ethical Requirements for Informed Consent for HIV Counseling and Testing

The principle of autonomy implies that a person should have some control over decisions regarding medical procedures he or she might undergo. A person's right to make these decisions is protected by a process called "informed consent." Mental health counselors may have opportunities to discuss informed consent with clients.

Procedures for Obtaining Informed Consent

1. Explain the test and inform the client of the pros and cons of testing.
2. Talk with the client to ensure that he or she understands the information.

3. Affirm confidentiality.

4. Stress the voluntary nature of consenting to the test.

A person must be informed of the risks and benefits of the proposed test or treatment before it is performed. This is the "informed" part of informed consent. Simply giving information is not enough. We must be assured that the client understands the information that we have provided. The client should always be given an opportunity to ask questions about the proposed test or treatment. It is also a good practice to ask the client to recount important points of information so you may evaluate the extent to which he or she understands the issues.

Because disclosure of HIV test information can lead to discrimination, it is important to affirm that this information will be kept confidential. However, one should not make unrealistic promises about confidentiality. For example, one should be honest about the fact that several members of the treatment team may have access to the test results. Finally, the client must consent to the test. Consent, to be valid, must be voluntary.

In most situations, informed consent for a medical procedure is not obtained in writing. However, in situations where the medical procedure is particularly serious or has potentially significant effects, such as an HIV test, informed consent is written and signed. This, however, does not remove the obligation to discuss the test with the client to ensure understanding.

There is a serious need to obtain informed consent for an HIV test because of the potentially devastating psychological effect of a positive result and because of the very real possibility of discrimination. The pretest counseling session, in which informed consent is obtained, also provides an excellent opportunity for client education. Information can be given about the ways HIV is transmitted, the means to prevent HIV transmission, and important facts about the HIV test. For example, it is important to know that the test may not pick up an infection acquired recently and that a negative result does not mean that the client is forever immune. Thus, while the primary purpose of obtaining informed consent is to safeguard a patient's autonomy, it also provides the opportunity to "do good" for the patient through education.

Confidentiality

Confidentiality is a fundamental aspect of medical and mental healthcare ethics. Clients expect that what they reveal to us in the course of care will be held in strict confidence. The ethical principle of responsibility requires that healthcare providers protect clients' rights to privacy.

Reasons to Maintain Confidentiality

- Personal privacy
- Therapeutic trust

Reasons to Breach Confidentiality

- The "duty to warn"
- The "need to know"
- The "duty to protect"

Most clients wish to maintain confidentiality, personal privacy, control, and all expressions of autonomy. Individuals in our society have a basic right to control what happens with their bodies. This principle underlies the process of informed consent, and it applies to personal control over health information. This, in itself, is reason enough for healthcare providers to maintain confidentiality.

Another reason to maintain confidentiality is that clients entrust private information to us; they trust us to be beneficent—to keep their best interest at heart. Without this trust, it is doubtful that many who need care would ever seek it. If healthcare providers commonly made public the information that clients wish to be kept private, then this would deter people from seeking care.

There are strong ethical reasons for maintaining confidentiality related to respect for persons and their privacy and to maintaining the trust that is implicit in the therapeutic relationship. Therefore, in cases where healthcare providers might want to breach confidentiality, there must be a strong and compelling reason.

When might it be appropriate to breach confidentiality? The clearest ethical indication occurs in cases where a known third person, for example, a sexual partner, may have been exposed to HIV, but the client refuses to notify the person. It is clearly the client's responsibility to notify known sexual and/or drug-use contacts. The client can do this personally or can do it anonymously through a contact tracing program.

If a client refuses to notify his or her contacts, and the healthcare provider is aware of the identity of the contacts, it is ethically defensible for the provider to breach confidentiality by warning known contacts of potential exposure. When a healthcare provider does this, he or she need not mention the client's name. This allows the provider to carry out what many call a "duty to warn," while at the same time trying to preserve confidentiality.

It is important to notify or warn past sex or needle-sharing partners of a client so that these contacts can seek counseling and testing. This will allow them to obtain appropriate treatment if they do test positive and to modify their behavior to prevent or reduce the spread of the infection to others. Again, every effort should be made to have the client carry out his or her responsibility before taking a step that could compromise confidentiality and lead to the perception of broken therapeutic trust.

This is a controversial issue. Before a staff member of a CMHC considers breaching confidentiality to notify a client contact, he or she should be aware of the state laws regarding this issue. States differ on the question of whether there is a legal duty to warn, apart from considerations of ethics. In some states, there is no legal duty to warn known contacts. Staff members should also be aware of protocols in their state and/or facility for breaching confidentiality. When protocols do permit a breach of confidentiality, it is often the prerogative and/or responsibility of the unit director. If a staff member becomes aware of a potentially infected partner of a client who is HIV-positive, the issue of breaching confidentiality should be referred to a supervisor.

Aside from the importance of warning potentially exposed third parties, some people cite a different reason for breaching confidentiality. They argue that there are situations where another individual has a "need to know" a client's HIV status, and that this person's "need to know" is great enough to justify breaching the client's confidentiality. Why would other individuals need to know a client's HIV status? The most pertinent reason is that these individuals are other healthcare providers whose "need to know" is tied to the delivery of appropriate healthcare. It is argued that if these individual healthcare providers are not made aware of the client's HIV status, then their diagnoses and treatment plans might be inappropriate. The principle of beneficence supports this particular "need to know" rationale.

Sharing a client's HIV information among providers directly involved in the client's care seems a natural extension of the traditional provider-client relationship, because healthcare more often involves multiple healthcare providers. However the "need to know" in a multiprovider context is still based on therapeutic trust; it is just expanded from a single provider to the other providers involved in the client's care. Each member of the care team has a responsibility to maintain the confidentiality of the client and, to avoid the perception of breached trust, clients should be told in advance that information is shared among treatment team members. Even so, this trust must be qualified; not all healthcare providers have a legitimate need to know. A person who works in a CMHC delivering meals to clients has no "need to know" a client's HIV status. A legitimate need to know can arise only among those providers who are involved in counseling and treating a client.

Others have claimed that they have a "need to know" based on the concept of self-preservation. They argue that they need to minimize their risk of HIV exposure and, therefore, need to know the client's HIV status so they can take extra precautions. It should be noted that these healthcare providers should already be taking universal precautions. There are no "extra precautions" recommended by the CDC. Often, these so-called extra precautions turn out to be a way that healthcare providers can avoid and discriminate against people identified as HIV-infected.

Still others may claim that they need to know clients' HIV status to protect those clients who are not HIV-infected. Once again, these protective measures often translate into providing different levels of care simply on the basis of HIV status, which may involve segregating HIV-infected clients from others. It has been suggested that HIV-infected clients should be kept from group activities because of fear that their presence would upset and, therefore, have a negative impact on the care of the noninfected clients. However, such practice is clearly discriminatory and violates the ethical principles guiding mental healthcare, especially the principle of justice. Group counseling sessions do not put anyone at risk for contracting HIV. To discriminate on this basis is without foundation.

There is appropriate concern, however, when a known HIV-infected client engages in behavior that puts other clients at risk. If an HIV-infected client exhibits threatening behavior toward other clients, such as attempting to bite, spit on, or initiate sex with them, then CMHC staff are justified in trying to protect other clients. Aside from these special situations, there are no justifications for sequestering an HIV-positive client or treating that client differently from others. While sexual activity and drug use are not permitted in CMHCs, all clients should be educated about the HIV risks associated with these behaviors. Through client education and procedures to minimize actual threats to clients, we can meet our duty to protect those persons under our care without discriminating against those who are infected with HIV.

Ethical Aspects of HIV Prevention and Education

Providing effective education to prevent the transmission of HIV is beneficent because it can help the client avoid HIV infection. This education also shows respect for individual autonomy because it empowers clients to make informed decisions. Effective education requires a basic tolerance for the beliefs of others, the recognition that people may make acceptable choices that differ from what one's own choice would be, and the commitment to talk about difficult topics in a frank and helpful manner.

Negative judgments of others may hinder mental healthcare providers' ability to serve clients' best interests. Counselors must keep any of their own discomfort about sexual behavior and drug use from interfering with their role as HIV prevention educators.

There are many reasons that talking about sex can be difficult. For many people, sex is personal and closely aligned with a loving relationship. The topic is not one that they discuss with "just anybody." Sex can also be difficult to talk about because sexual practices differ from individual to individual. Some practices might seem "out of the ordinary," or perhaps even disgusting, to some people. Last, sex can be difficult to talk about because some types of sexual behavior might be at odds with one's moral or religious convictions. It is difficult to speak in a nonjudgmental way about a type of sexual act that one feels is wrong or sinful.

However, it is important to talk about sex in the context of HIV. Former Surgeon General C. Everett Koop stated that the only weapon available against the AIDS epidemic is education. Because HIV is transmitted sexually, it is necessary to educate people about preventing sexual transmission. Furthermore, effective education in this context means education that leads to behavioral change. Thus, it is necessary to talk in easily understood terms and to present advice that is relevant and feasible for clients to follow.

The most effective way to offer AIDS education is to provide facts about the sexual transmission of HIV and present a range of options regarding prevention. Consider the following range of options:

Options Regarding Sex

- Abstinence from sex
- Mutual monogamy with an uninfected partner
- Safer sex: nonpenetrative sexual contact
- Safer sex: intercourse with barrier protection (e.g., condoms)

Sex is an important aspect of life, and, for many people, abstinence may not be a desirable or realistic option. If abstinence is the only option presented, then individuals who are not abstinent may not protect themselves in other ways simply because they have not learned how to have safer sex. Providing a range of options empowers people to protect themselves against HIV in the way most beneficial for them. In this context, it is helpful to discuss with the client that the use of alcohol and drugs decreases a person's ability to make responsible decisions about sex. Helping the client to recognize this, and to change behavior accordingly, is a further component of the principle of respect for autonomy, since these interventions enhance the client's ability to control his or her own life.

This reasoning holds true for injection drug use also. Most clinicians would agree that not using injectable drugs is the best option, but, for some clients, this might be unrealistic given their current situation. Thus, to prevent HIV transmission, the problems arising from sharing needles and procedures for cleaning needles, syringes, and drug paraphernalia should be discussed (Gostin, Lazzarini, Jones, and Flaherty, 1997). Offering the following range of options regarding drug use is appropriate:

Options Regarding Drug Use

- Abstain from drug use.
- If you do use drugs, do not share needles, syringes, and paraphernalia.
- If you must share, clean the needles and syringes with bleach.

Community mental health center workers may feel they are being unethical by presenting a range of options regarding possible "immoral" behavior. Our judgments as counselors about the best or most moral choice may not coincide with the choices clients make. The ethical principle of autonomy is relevant here. As healthcare providers, we recognize that clients have the right to make choices about their bodies. Thus, while we may encourage what we feel to be the "best" option, choosing not to provide all the information limits the client's freedom to make choices. Clients are more likely to choose to protect themselves if they have a choice among several "safer" options.

Conclusion

The HIV epidemic has presented healthcare providers with new challenges, especially in the area of ethics. There are four ethical principles that guide the practice of mental healthcare: beneficence, autonomy, justice, and responsibility. These principles help us understand attitudinal barriers to delivering competent and compassionate mental healthcare to HIV-infected clients. These principles also guide our approach to issues involving informed consent, HIV testing, confidentiality, and prevention education. These principles not only provide a useful framework for thinking about ethical issues, but they can also serve as tools to help us work through ethical problems that occur in CMHCs.

Review Questions

1. How does "beneficence," or doing good, pertain to the treatment of clients?

2. Name the components of informed consent for an HIV test.

3. What are the sexual options that should be discussed with a client when educating him or her about preventing sexual transmission of HIV?

4. How might a caregiver build a relationship of therapeutic trust with a client?

5. How do negative attitudes among caregivers about life-styles such as homosexuality affect the quality of care received by a client with HIV disease?

References and Suggested Readings

Annas, G.J. (1988). Not saints, but healers: The legal duties of health care professionals in the AIDS epidemic. *American Journal of Public Health, 78,* 844–849.

Beauchamp, T.L. & Childress, J.F. (1994). *Principles of Biomedical Ethics.* New York: Oxford University Press.

Bowers, S.A. (1991). The Americans with Disabilities Act. *American Journal of Orthodontics and Dentofacial Orthopedics, 100,* 290–292.

Brown, M.L. (1987). AIDS and ethics: Concerns and considerations. *Oncology Nursing Forum, 14,* 69–73.

Cameron, M.E., Chrisham, P., & Lewis, D.E. (1994). The content of ethical problems experienced by persons with AIDS. *Journal of the Association of Nurses in AIDS Care, 5,* 32–42.

Chaisson, R.E., Keruly, J.C., & Moore, R.D. (1995). Race, sex, drug use and progression of human immunodeficiency virus disease. *New England Journal of Medicine, 333,* 751–756.

Cochran, S.D., & Mays, V.M. (1989). Women and AIDS-related concerns. *American Psychologist, 44*(3), 529–535.

Council on Ethical and Judicial Affairs. (1988). Ethical issues involved in the growing AIDS crisis. *Journal of the American Medical Association, 259,* 1360–1361.

Dannenberg, A.L., McNeil, J.G., Brundage, J.F., & Brookmeyer, R. (1996). Suicide and HIV infection. *Journal of the American Medical Association, 276*(21), 1743–1746.

Deeks, S.G., Smith, M., Holodniy, M., & Kahn, J.O. (1997). HIV-1 protease inhibitors. *Journal of the American Medical Association, 277*(2), 145–153.

Gillon, R. (Ed.) (1994). *Principles of Healthcare Ethics.* London: John Wiley & Sons.

Gordin, F.M., Willoughby, A.D., Levine, L.A., Gurel, L., & Neill, K.M. (1987). Knowledge of AIDS among hospital workers: Behavioral correlates and consequences. *AIDS, 1,* 183–188.

Gostin, L.O., Lazzarini, Z., Jones, T.S., & Flaherty, K. (1997). Prevention of HIV/AIDS and other blood-borne diseases among injection drug users. *Journal of the American Medical Association, 277*(1), 53–62.

Green, S.A. (1995). The ethical limits of confidentiality in the therapeutic relationship. *General Hospital Psychiatry, 17,* 80–84.

Halperin, E.C. (1988). The right to privacy and the duty to protect. *Southern Medical Journal, 81,* 1286–1290.

Hoffman, B.F., Arthurs, K., Lunn, S., Meyers, L., Trimnell J., & Farcnik, K. (1989). AIDS: Clinical and ethical issues on a psychiatric unit. *Canadian Journal of Psychiatry—Revue Canadienne De Psychiatrie, 34,* 847–852.

Kadzielski, M.A. (1989). Fighting fear with facts: Understanding the ethical and legal aspects of AIDS. *Today's OR-Nurse, 11,* 33–37.

Kelly, J.A., St. Lawrence, J.S., Brasfield, T.L, Lemke, A., Amidei, T., McNeill, C., Hood, H.V., Smith, J.E., & Kilgore, H. (1990). Psychological factors that predict AIDS high-risk versus AIDS precautionary behavior. *Journal of Consulting and Clinical Psychology, 1,* 117–120.

Kelly, J.A., St. Lawrence, J.S., Smith, S., Jr., Hood, H.V., & Cook, D.J. (1987). Stigmatization of AIDS patients by physicians. *American Journal of Public Health, 77,* 789–791.

Mariner, W.K. (1995). AIDS phobia, public health warnings, and lawsuits: Deterring harm or rewarding ignorance. *American Journal of Public Health, 85,* 1562–1568.

McKinnon, M.D., Insall, C., Gooch, C.D., & Cockcroft, A. (1990). Knowledge and attitudes of health care workers about AIDS and HIV infection before and after distribution of an educational booklet. *Journal of the Society of Occupational Medicine, 40,* 15–18.

Murphy, T.F., & Walters, L. (1994). The moral significance of AIDS. *Journal of Medicine and Philosophy, 19,* 519–524.

Pellegrino, E.D. (1989). HIV infection and the ethics of clinical care. *Journal of Legal Medicine, 10,* 29–46.

Polan, H.J., Hellerstein, D., & Amchin, J. (1985). Impact of AIDS-related cases on an inpatient therapeutic milieu. *Hospital and Community Psychiatry, 36,* 173–176.

Rothenberg, K.H., & Paskey, S.T. (1995). The risk of domestic violence and women with HIV infection: Implications for partner notification, public policy, and the law. *American Journal of Public Health, 85,* 1569–1576.

Searight, H.R., & Pound, P. (1994). The HIV-positive psychiatric patient and the duty to protect: Ethical and legal issues. *International Journal of Psychiatric Medicine, 24,* 259–270.

Strax, T.E. (1994). Ethical issues of treating patients with AIDS in a rehabilitation setting. *American Journal of Physical Medicine and Rehabilitation, 73,* 293–295.

Touhey, J.F. (1995). Moving from autonomy to responsibility in HIV-related healthcare. *Cambridge Quarterly of Healthcare Ethics, 4*(1), 64–70.

Voelker, R. (1995). AIDS and human rights. *Journal of the American Medical Association, 274*(20), 1577.

Wallack, J.J. (1991). AIDS and the health care professional: Evolving attitudes and strategies to effect change. *Psychiatric Medicine, 9,* 483–501.

Wertz, D.C., Sorenson, J.R., Liebling, L., Kessler, L., & Heeren, T.C. (1987). Knowledge and attitudes of AIDS health care providers before and after education programs. *Public Health Reports, 102,* 248–254.

Part II

Understanding HIV Healthcare

Chapter 5

The Clinician's Role in Early Detection of HIV

Michael D. Knox, Ph.D., and
Charles F. Clark, M.D., M.P.H.

Overview

This chapter discusses the importance of early detection of HIV, the clinician's role, and indications of HIV infection. Community mental health center (CMHC) staff are encouraged to become proactive in recognizing clients who are at risk of HIV disease. CMHCs can play an important role in early detection and referral. This chapter draws on work by Knox and Clark (1991), published in the *Journal of Mental Health Administration.*

Learning Objectives

1. To state the benefits of early detection of HIV.

2. To recognize symptoms of HIV disease from a client history and to observe for neuropsychological and physical signs of HIV disease.

3. To make appropriate referrals for counseling, testing, and medical and support services for HIV-infected clients.

4. To improve the clinician's ability to respond to HIV-infected clients' needs.

Outline

I. Need for Early Detection
   A. Early concerns about negative effects of HIV testing
   B. Individual benefits of early detection
      1. Increased life expectancy
      2. Prompt medical care
         a. Access to HIV treatment drugs
         b. Avoidance of medical hazards
      3. Protection of partners and other people
      4. Opportunity to make decisions about having children
      5. Improved quality of life through alterations in life-style
      6. Opportunity to resolve personal beliefs about life and death
      7. Life planning
   C. Institutional benefits of early detection
      1. Identify vulnerable special populations
      2. Anticipate service needs
      3. Planning

II. Recognizing the Indicators of HIV Infection through Early Screening
   A. Client history
   B. Neuropsychological signs of infection
   C. Observing physical signs of infection
   D. Recognizing related infections

III. Role of Community Mental Health Centers in Referring Clients for Testing
   A. Outpatients
   B. Inpatients

IV. Conclusion

Need for Early Detection

Early detection of HIV disease has become increasingly important to the physical and mental health of the individual. CMHC staff can play an important role in early detection. Screening for exposure to HIV should become a standard part of client assessment.

Early Concerns about Negative Effects of HIV Detection

In the early years of the HIV/AIDS epidemic, many people thought that, since no medical treatments were available, knowing one's HIV status might do more harm than good. A number of possible negative effects of early identification of HIV disease were suggested.

Possible Negative Effects of Knowing HIV Status

- Increased psychological stress for clients and CMHC staff
- Discrimination against persons with HIV infection
- Avoidance by mental health workers or medical workers of HIV-positive persons
- Liability of the agency if confidentiality was breached
- Financial obligation of agencies to treat HIV-infected persons
- Liability to inform spouses and/or lovers of HIV-infected persons
- Mandatory obligation to offer treatment

The first three concerns: increased psychological stress, discrimination, and avoidance by healthcare workers are concerns about the impact on a client of learning his or her HIV status. The other concerns are about the impact that early detection might have on a mental health agency and its staff. In fact, CMHC clinicians have reported discomfort in working with HIV-infected persons. Research has demonstrated (Dow and Knox, 1991) that many center treatment staff would prefer to avoid HIV-infected clients and some staff would actively avoid working with these persons. It is important that CMHC staff become comfortable working with HIV-infected persons and learn more about the importance of recognizing and treating HIV disease as early in the disease process as possible. It is also important that staff understand that early detection benefits both the client and the agency.

Individual Benefits of Early Detection

As the health professions have learned more about HIV disease, the benefits of early detection have come to outweigh the possible negative effects. It is time to overcome any remaining antitesting, antidiagnosis bias in public mental health settings. Today, early detection can bring many positive benefits to HIV-infected persons. It can also improve the quality of care offered by staffs of CMHCs.

Benefits of Early Detection of HIV

- Increased life expectancy
- Prompt medical care
- Access to HIV treatment drugs
- Avoidance of medical hazards
- Protection of partners and other people
- Opportunity to make decisions about having children
- Reduced HIV transmission to offspring
- Improved quality of life through alterations in life-style
- Resolution of personal beliefs about life and death
- Life planning

For an individual client, early detection can bring many of the above benefits.

Increased Life Expectancy

Many people who are HIV-infected may be asymptomatic for many years. As more treatments are developed, the length of survival is increasing. If a person's immune status is monitored medically and drug treatments are begun at the appropriate times, life expectancy increases.

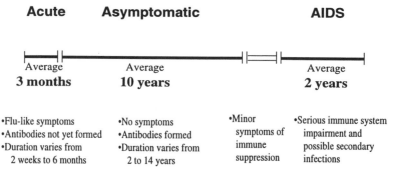

FIGURE 5.1 Progression of HIV Disease

The diagram shown above depicts the progression of HIV and AIDS. People who are exposed to HIV may develop a flulike illness during the acute phase. During this phase, since antibodies are just beginning to be formed, HIV testing may be negative. People then enter a long period in which they are asymptomatic, although some may experience swelling of the lymph glands. HIV antibodies are present so that testing is effective. Once AIDS symptoms appear, the survival time from the diagnosis of AIDS to death has averaged two years, but long survivals do occur with good healthcare.

We do not know when a cure for HIV disease will be found; it could be next year or far into the future. Drugs are currently available to slow the progression of the disease, and every person with HIV disease can look forward to a possible cure before the disease moves into its final stages. Suggesting that an HIV-infected person hope for more effective treatments, without creating false expectations, can be a sustaining factor to combat a sense of hopelessness.

Prompt Medical Care

The asymptomatic period of the disease may be prolonged with prompt medical care.

Access to HIV Treatment Drugs. Prompt and appropriate medical care includes treatment with an increasing number of Food and Drug Administration (FDA) approved drugs, as discussed in Chapter 7, "Medical Management." Many of these inhibit viral replication and are thought to slow the progression of HIV infection, thus delaying the onset of AIDS. While these drugs are helping many persons with HIV, they are not cures for the disease. A cure would mean that the virus could be eliminated from the patient. Research is focused on finding such a cure, but none exists yet.

These drugs, and various prophylactic drugs against opportunistic infections, form the basis of a growing array of medical options for prolonging and improving the quality of the lives of persons with HIV disease. It is important for HIV-infected clients to be identified, so that they can be provided with primary medical care on an ongoing basis and the infections that constitute the syndrome can be prevented or treated at the earliest stages.

Avoidance of Medical Hazards. Early diagnosis also enables persons who are HIV-infected to avoid routine medical procedures that may be dangerous to them. Except under special circumstances, HIV-infected persons should not accept live-virus vaccines. They should avoid exposure to infectious diseases.

HIV-positive persons should obtain prompt medical attention for any fever, night sweats, or other symptoms suggestive of an infection. It is hypothesized that viral and bacterial infections may "turn on" production of HIV and hasten the development of AIDS. Infectious agents such as syphilis, herpes, tuberculosis, hepatitis B, and measles may be more severe in an HIV-infected person and may require special medical attention.

Protection of Partners and Other People

Knowledge of one's HIV status allows an individual to adopt safer sex practices that will protect a partner or spouse. Individuals can also inform past partners so that those people may learn their own HIV status. Knowledge of one's HIV status gives a person the opportunity and responsibility to protect other people by refraining from donating blood, semen, or body organs to medical facilities.

Opportunity to Make Decisions about Having Children

Both women and men who know their HIV status can make informed decisions about whether to have children. Women who are HIV-infected have an opportunity to consider the potential effect of pregnancy on their HIV infection. Women also need to consider that some children born to HIV-positive mothers are born infected with the virus. All children carry their mother's antibodies and, therefore, initially will test HIV-positive if the mother is. The antibodies will clear by the age of two for most of the children, but 15–30 percent (Centers for Disease Control and Prevention, 1995) will remain positive, as they are actually infected with HIV disease. Zidovudine (AZT), when given to previously untreated mothers and their offspring, can reduce the transmission rate by 67 percent. This is another important reason for early HIV detection.

The prognosis for HIV-infected children is bimodal. Approximately 25 percent will have a mean survival of two years and 75 percent will have a mean survival of eight years.

Women who are considering pregnancy through artificial insemination should consider the risk of sperm donors being HIV-positive and take steps to assure their protection. Sperm banks generally test donors and then freeze sperm until the donor is retested six months later.

Men who are HIV-positive and are partners with women must consider the danger of unprotected sexual intercourse to their partners and future children. Also, many children born uninfected to mothers who are infected are likely to be left as orphans early in life.

Improved Quality of Life through Alterations in Life-style

It is never too late to adopt positive, health-promoting behaviors. The following life-style changes can improve the quality of life for a person with HIV.

Alter Life-style to Improve the Quality of Life

DO

- Reduce stress.
- Enter drug and alcohol treatment.
- Seek mental health counseling.

- Practice good nutrition and safe food preparation.
- Keep practicing safer sex.
- Practice good hygiene around pets.
- Take protective measures when visiting clinics and hospitals.

DON'T

- Be a workaholic.
- Smoke cigarettes.
- Inject drugs.
- Drink alcohol.
- Ignore other people's infections.

Altering one's life-style in ways that may improve immune system functioning may include stress reduction programs, drug or alcohol recovery programs, and mental health counseling. An HIV-infected individual may take advantage of good nutrition to boost the immune system's ability to fight AIDS-related diseases.

A person with HIV disease can engage in safe behaviors that protect oneself and others from further infection. For example, persons who are HIV-positive and are having sexual relations with other HIV-infected persons can still protect themselves from reinfection by different HIV strains by using safer sex techniques.

People can also avoid exposing themselves to other hazards to their immune systems. They may change their living environment to cut down on exposure to disease from pets, adopt safer food handling practices, and be careful to avoid people with infectious conditions. For example, sitting in a medical clinic waiting room with sick people or visiting hospitals may be dangerous for the health of HIV-positive people. The list of "don'ts" includes behavior that may depress the immune system. Avoiding these practices: working too hard, smoking, using drugs or alcohol, and exposing oneself to infections may prolong life.

Opportunity to Resolve Personal Beliefs about Life and Death

For many HIV-infected persons, and especially for persons with AIDS, the period following a diagnosis of a fatal disease is a time to examine their personal philosophies and beliefs. Counseling, programs of meditation, study groups, and support groups can offer valuable opportunities for self-examination and resolution of issues related to life and death. Some persons with AIDS have been sustained through their illness by their spiritual beliefs or participation in healing rituals or formal religion.

Life Planning

Persons infected with HIV need time to plan their remaining lives. Planning includes an individual's understanding of where on the continuum of HIV/AIDS he or she is at the time of diagnosis and then making short-range and long-range plans. Persons who are asymptomatic may realign long-range goals. A person may want time to resolve family issues. As a person's disease progresses to AIDS, he or she may need time to make arrangements for care of dependents and pets. Arranging for intermediate and terminal care; creating a will, living will, and estate arrangements; and making funeral and memorial decisions are all part of life planning. (See Chapter 14, "Preparing for Death.")

Institutional Benefits of Early Detection

Community mental health centers, state psychiatric hospitals, and other public mental health facilities will be seeing an increasing number of HIV-infected clients. Early detection of the HIV status of these clients has several benefits.

Institutional Benefits of Early Detection

- Identifying vulnerable special populations
- Anticipating service needs
- Planning

Early HIV counseling and testing of agency clients allows institutions to identify special populations that are vulnerable to HIV infection. For example, persons with serious and persistent mental illness are a special at-risk group often characterized by poor impulse control, impaired judgment, sexual promiscuity, and drug use. (See Chapter 17, "Treating Persons with Serious and Persistent Mental Illness.")

Early detection allows an institution to anticipate future service and treatment needs for HIV-infected clients. Advance planning also allows time to secure needed sources of revenue, such as government or third-party payors, and to allocate resources appropriately.

Recognizing the Indicators of HIV Infection through Early Screening

The purpose of early screening for HIV infection is to become proactive in linking clients who are HIV-infected to services. CMHC staff may be the first care providers to see indications of HIV infection. Many HIV-infected clients show symptoms of central nervous system damage, which may present as a psychiatric illness. The Centers for Disease Control and Prevention (CDC) definition of AIDS includes: encephalopathy, wasting syndrome, and constitutional symptoms. Approximately 15 percent of individuals receive a diagnosis of AIDS on the basis of neurological disease. The onset of dementia is now recognized as the beginning manifestation of HIV encephalopathy. For CMHC staff, observing neuropsychological and physical signs of infection is an important part of HIV screening. The client's history may disclose risk activity, which may prompt HIV testing and early detection.

Taking the steps listed below should become a routine part of client assessment for HIV disease.

Assessing Clients for Referral to HIV Counseling and Testing

- Take a thorough sexual and substance abuse history.
- Ask about recent health problems suggestive of HIV.
- Assess neuropsychological symptoms.
- Notice physical signs that may indicate HIV.

Client History

The client history is the most important indicator of possible exposure to HIV. HIV screening should become a standard part of taking a client history. A client's social, sexual, or drug use history may indicate behaviors that carry a high risk of infection. The primary risk groups in this country continue to be men who have sex with other men, and injecting drug users or sexual partners of past or current injecting drug users. Involvement with crack cocaine is a significant risk factor, especially for women. Clients with mental illness who may have poor impulse control are at special risk of infection. Even clients with low levels of sexual activity, but with more than one partner, may be at risk because a single occurrence of sexual intercourse may result in HIV infection. Emerging groups with heterosexual intercourse as a primary risk factor include women, adolescents, and the elderly.

Diagnosing AIDS in the elderly is problematic because many clinicians fail to recognize AIDS as a possibility. HIV infection is often not considered by staff until late in the course of illness. Research has shown that about 10 percent of elderly Americans have at least one risk factor for HIV infection. Very few of these persons use condoms during sex or have undergone HIV testing.

A client's history should also include asking questions about physical symptoms consistent with HIV infection. These may include:

Physical Symptoms Related to HIV Infection That May Be Revealed in a Client's History

- Unexplained weight loss
- Persistent diarrhea
- Night sweats
- Recurrent fever
- Swollen glands
- Recurrent or chronic oral infections
- Recurrent vaginal infections
- Decreasing vision with eye pain
- Bleeding gums
- Persistent mouth sores
- Pain on swallowing
- Recent onset of headaches
- Easy tiring
- Irritability
- Loss of interest in friends and usual activities

Once these general health problems are covered in the client history, an evaluation of mental status can be made.

Neuropsychological Signs of Infection

"Mental" symptoms may precede the development of the opportunistic infections associated with AIDS. An infected person may have a single complaint or a constellation of symptoms.

Neuropsychological Signs of Infection

- Slowed thinking

- Decreased memory
- Sleep disturbance
- Poor appetite
- Weight loss
- Tiredness
- Lethargy
- Apathy
- Organic psychosis
- Agitation
- Confusion

The first eight common symptoms may easily be mistaken for depression. Clients may also present with other less common symptoms such as organic psychosis, agitation, or confusion. In elderly clients it is often difficult to determine if dementia is caused by HIV. Studies show a beneficial effect of certain antiretroviral treatments on mental functioning. Appropriate client care requires an early diagnosis. Clients and their families may seek help at a CMHC because they observe symptoms that are traditionally cared for in a mental health setting. It is the responsibility of CMHC staff to know that the symptoms listed above may indicate HIV infection so that proper testing and diagnosis can be accomplished. (See Chapter 9, "Neuropsychological Functioning in HIV Disease.")

Observing Physical Signs of Infection

Even with no neuropsychological symptoms, CMHC staff should be alert to observable physical signs in their clients. Nonmedical clinical staff should be trained to recognize physical signs that can be directly observed during an interview or that a client reports. These conditions could include the following:

Physical Signs of HIV Infection

- Severe dandruff
- Acne
- Oral thrush (candidiasis)
- Skin rashes

- Purplish spots
- Facial warts
- Ill-fitting clothes from weight loss
- Unsteady gait
- Persistent cold sores
- Persistent sinus infection

Note: Symptoms are subjectively reported while signs are objectively observed.

Although these conditions do not necessarily mean that a person is infected with HIV, they are present with increased frequency in patients with HIV.

Recognizing Related Infections

Some physical conditions are suggestive of HIV infection. Community mental healthcare providers should be aware of the following manifestations of infections that often coexist with HIV infection and refer clients for medical evaluation.

Infections that May Coexist with HIV Disease

- Herpes—weeping skin lesions
- Hepatitis B—nausea and yellow eyes
- Tuberculosis—productive cough, night sweats, and weight loss
- Shingles—angry painful rash
- Syphilis—painless ulcer or generalized rash

Role of Community Mental Health Centers in Referring Clients for Testing

After a thorough screening, the CMHC staff role in early detection includes encouraging clients who have a likelihood of HIV infection to be tested. It is important to listen to a client's concerns and to evaluate his or her readiness for testing before the referral is made. One of the important functions of CMHC counselors is to link clients to the network of services they will need. Procedures will differ for outpatient and inpatient mental health clients.

Outpatients

Outpatient testing in the community is a more normalizing experience and may result in better coordination of services for the client in the event of a positive test result. Outpatients should be referred, and perhaps even accompanied by a case worker, to a public health clinic. An outpatient referred through the public health system may be offered support groups, medical clinic visits, public health counseling, and other services not available at the CMHC. Clients should be asked to bring their test results back to the CMHC or to sign a consent form so that the information can be released to the primary therapist or case manager. Clients may panic while waiting for results, so counselors serve a supportive role during the waiting period. The steps in the outpatient referral process are:

Steps in Referral Process

Step 1. Have the primary therapist or case manager determine the risk of HIV infection.

Step 2. Discuss the need for testing with client.

> Discuss anonymous or confidential testing options.
>
> Assess readiness for testing.
>
> Obtain informed consent to release results to CMHC.
>
> Introduce preventive concepts.

Step 3. Refer to private physician, public health clinic, or other local testing sites.

Step 4. Provide follow-up counseling.

> Reinforce preventive education messages.
>
> Monitor symptoms.
>
> Monitor compliance with infection control measures.
>
> Coordinate availability and use of support services.
>
> Encourage compliance with medical regimen.

It is important to refer clients for testing who may be at low risk for HIV but who are worried about being infected. Receiving negative results may reassure these clients and relieve some of their anxiety about their health status.

Inpatients

Inpatient counseling and testing can be completed while a client is in the hospital so that results are available during treatment. Appropriate pretest and posttest counseling is essential following protocols that may be required by state government or agency policy.

During the time an inpatient is waiting for results, unit staff may notice behavior change associated with anxiety. Support through anxiety management techniques may be helpful. The steps in the inpatient referral process are:

Steps in Referral Process

Step 1. After intake, have the primary therapist or case manager refer the client for in-house pretest counseling, testing, and posttest counseling.

Step 2. Provide follow-up counseling.

Reinforce preventive education messages.

Monitor symptoms.

Monitor compliance with infection control measures.

Coordinate availability and use of support services.

Encourage compliance with medical regimen.

Conclusion

Early detection of HIV disease allows a client to obtain appropriate medical and mental healthcare, avoid infection, make informed reproductive decisions, and behave responsibly so as not to infect others. Testing provides the opportunity for a client to receive preventive education and guidance for limiting further transmission of the disease. Primary therapists and case managers can repeat the educational message frequently; monitor signs, symptoms, and compliance with infection control measures; and coordinate necessary health, mental health, and social services. CMHCs must be able to identify affected clients, anticipate service needs, and provide a variety of services to meet the needs of HIV-infected clientele.

Review Questions

1. What are the benefits of early detection of HIV disease?

2. What are five physical signs of possible HIV infection?

3. Are unexplained weight loss and recurrent fevers *always* indicators of HIV disease?

4. Identify the signs of neuropsychological impairment from HIV disease.

5. Describe how a CMHC can best serve clients with HIV disease.

References and Suggested Readings

Atkinson, J.H., & Grant, I. (1994). Natural history of neuropsychiatric manifestations of HIV disease. *The Psychiatric Clinics of North America, 17*(1), 17–33.

Bigger, R.J., Pahwa S., Minkoff, H., Mendes, H., Willoughby, A., Landesman, S., & Goedert, J.J. (1989). Immunosuppression in pregnant women infected with human immuno-deficiency virus. *American Journal of Obstetrics and Gynecology, 161,* 1239–1244.

Blanche, S., Rouzioux, C., Moscato, M.L., Veber, F., Mayaux, M.J., Jacomet, C., Tricoire, J., Deville, A., Vial, M., Firtion, G., De Crepy, A., Douard, D., Robin, M., Courpotin, C., Ciraru-Vigneron, N., Le Deist, F., Griscelli, C., & the HIV Infection in Newborns French Collaborative Study Group (1989). A prospective study of infants born to women seroposi-tive for human immunodeficiency virus Type 1: HIV Infection in Newborns French Collaborative Study Group. *New England Journal of Medicine, 320,* 1643–1648.

Bono, G., Zandrini, C., Brusta, R., Sinforiani, E., Barbarini, G., & Mogglia, A. (1990). Neuropsychological and neurophysiological abnormalities in HIV infection: Their rele-vance and predictive value. *Acta Neurologica, 12*(1), 4–8.

Centers for Disease Control and Prevention. (1995). U.S. Public Health Service recommenda-tions for HIV counseling and voluntary testing for pregnant women. *Morbidity and Mortality Weekly Report, 44*(No. RR-7).

Detmer, W.M., & Lu, F.G. (1986). Neuropsychiatric complications of AIDS: A literature review. *International Journal of Psychiatry in Medicine, 16*(1), 21–29.

Dow, M.G., & Knox, M.D. (1991). Mental health and substance abuse staff: HIV/AIDS knowl-edge and attitudes. *AIDS Care, 3*(1), 75–87.

Dow, M.G., Knox, M.D., & Cotton, D.A. (1989). Administrative challenges to working with HIV-positive clients: Experiences of mental health and substance abuse program directors in Florida. *Journal of Mental Health Administration, 16*(2), 80–90.

Fernandez, F. (1990). Psychopharmacological interventions in HIV infections. *New Directions for Mental Health Services, 48,* 43–53.

Horwath, E., Kramer, M., Cournos, F., Empfield, M., & Gewirtz, G. (1989). Clinical presenta-tions of AIDS and HIV infection in state psychiatric facilities. *Hospital and Community Psychiatry, 40,* 502–506.

Jewett, J.F., & Hecht, F.M. (1993). Preventative health care for adults with HIV infection. *Journal of the American Medical Association, 269*(9), 1144–1153.

Kieburtz, K.D., Ketonen, L., Zettelmaier, A., Kido, D., Caine, E.D., & Simon, J.H. (1990). Magnetic resonance imaging findings in HIV cognitive impairment. *Archives of Neurology, 47,* 643–645.

Knox, M.D. (1989). Community mental health's role in the AIDS crisis. *Community Mental Health Journal, 25*(3), 185–196.

Knox, M.D., Boaz, T.L., Friedrich, M.A., & Dow, M.G. (1994). HIV risk factors for persons with serious mental illness. *Community Mental Health Journal, 30*(6), 551–563.

Knox, M.D., & Clark, C.F. (1991). Early HIV detection: A community mental health role. *Journal of Mental Health Administration, 18*(1), 21–26.

Knox, M.D., Friedrich, M.A., Gaies, J.S., & Achenbach, K. (1994). Training HIV Specialists for Community Mental Health. *Community Mental Health Journal, 30*(4), 405–413.

Marotta, R., & Perry, S. (1989). Early neuropsychological dysfunction caused by human immunodeficiency virus. *Journal of Neuropsychiatry and Clinic Neurosciences, 1*(3), 225–235.

Pratt, R.D., Hatch, R., Dankner, W.M., & Spector, S.A. (1993). Pediatric human immunodeficiency virus infection in a low seroprevalence area. *Pediatric Infectious Disease Journal, 12*(4), 304–310.

Rabkin, J.G., Williams, J.B., Neugebauer, R., Remien, R.H., & Goetz, R. (1990). Maintenance of hope in HIV-spectrum homosexual men. *American Journal of Psychiatry, 147,* 1322–1326.

Redfield, R.R., Wright, D.C., James, W.D., Jones, T.S., Brown, C., & Burke, D.S. (1989). Disseminated vaccine in a military recruit with human immunodeficiency virus (HIV) disease. *New England Journal of Medicine, 316,* 673–676.

Scott, G.B., Hutto, C., Makuch, R.W., Mastrucci, M.T., O'Conner, T., Mitchell, C.D., Trapido, E.J., & Parks, W.P. (1989). Survival in children with perinatally acquired human immunodeficiency virus Type 1 infection. *New England Journal of Medicine, 321,* 1791–1796.

Sidtis, J.J. & Price, R.W. (1990). Early HIV-1 infection and the AIDS dementia complex. *Neurology, 40*(2), 323–326.

Stall, R. & Catania, J. (1994). AIDS risk behaviors among late middle-aged and elderly Americans. The National AIDS Behavioral Surveys. *Archives of Internal Medicine, 154*(1), 57–63.

Wright, E., Fitzgerald, A., Risi, G., & Marier, R. (1989). AIDS: Diagnosing educational needs of health care professionals. *International Conference on AIDS V,* Abstract E.609.

Chapter 6

■ **HIV Transmission in Healthcare Settings and Infection Control for Healthcare Workers**

Barbara Russell, R.N., C.I.C., A.C.R.N., M.P.H.

Overview

This chapter focuses on the risk and prevention of HIV transmission in healthcare facilities, including community mental health centers (CMHCs). The material includes a summary of the Centers for Disease Control and Prevention's (CDC) studies of healthcare workers' risk of exposure to HIV in the workplace. Procedures for implementing the CDC universal precautions and Occupational Safety and Health Administration (OSHA) standards of protection are reviewed. This review is followed by a presentation of steps individuals and agencies should take in managing exposure, if it does occur.

Learning Objectives

1. To cite the primary mode of HIV transmission from patient-to-healthcare worker.

2. To list at least three applications of the CDC universal precautions to protect patients and healthcare workers.

3. To understand an employer's obligations for testing, clinical management, and treatment of an HIV-infected healthcare worker.

Outline

I. Healthcare Workers' Risk of HIV Infection

    A. Review of CDC study of healthcare workers

    B. Primary risk linked to large-bore needles in direct contact with blood

    C. Review of cases reported to CDC

II. Patients'/Clients' Risk of Acquiring HIV Infection in Healthcare Settings

    A. Healthcare worker-to-patient transmission

    B. Patient-to-patient transmission

III. Preventing Workplace Exposure by Adhering to CDC Universal Precautions and OSHA Guidelines

    A. Procedures for disposing of sharp instruments after use

    B. Personal precautions

        1. Avoid direct contact with blood or body fluids

        2. Use of personal protective equipment

    C. Handling instruments and equipment

IV. Management of an Exposure

V. Conclusion

Healthcare Workers' Risk of Infection

Review of CDC Study of Healthcare Workers

Through ongoing studies, the CDC and other researchers have estimated the risk to a healthcare worker of acquiring HIV through an occupational exposure is approximately 0.3 percent. To put this in perspective, a healthcare worker who has never had hepatitis B disease or the hepatitis B vaccine has a 6 percent to 30 percent risk of acquiring the hepatitis virus through occupational exposure.

An occupational exposure is defined as receiving a percutaneous injury (i.e., an injury through the skin by a needle or sharp object) or a mucocutaneous exposure from an infected individual. A mucocutaneous exposure is the entry of an infected person's blood or body fluid into the eyes, nose, mouth, or an open, unprotected cut of another person. Clearly, occupational exposures are not likely to occur to nonmedical staff of CMHCs.

Primary Risk Linked to Large-Bore Needles in Direct Contact with Blood

Specific data collected by the CDC through December 1996 indicate that 52 healthcare workers in the United States have been fully documented to have acquired HIV through occupational exposure (Table 6.1).

TABLE 6.1 Fifty-two Cases of Occupationally Acquired HIV

| Type of Exposure | | | |
Percutaneous	Mucocutaneous	Both	Unknown
45 (86%)	5 (10%)	1 (2%)	1 (2%)

| Personnel Involved | | | | |
Nurses	Clinical Lab Workers	Physicians	Other	Mental Health Workers
21	19	6	6	0

Current CDC data indicate that the most frequent cause of occupational transmission is an injury from a large-bore, 16 to 18 gauge, blood-contaminated needle that was placed directly in a vein or artery of a source patient with terminal AIDS illness.

"Fully documented" means that the injured worker had an HIV antibody test done close to the time of the exposure which was negative and subsequently, within six months after the injury, developed a positive HIV antibody test. Six months is currently considered the "window period" for seroconversion after exposure to HIV. The worker is usually tested at six weeks, three months, and six months following the initial injury and, if still negative at six months, is told that no HIV transmission has occurred.

CDC has data on another 111 cases listed as "likely" cases of HIV transmission in the workplace. None of the occupationally acquired cases have occurred in mental health workers. Since the major risk is from needlestick injuries, nurses and laboratory workers incur most of the injuries. Most mental health workers have no, or extremely limited, contact with these sharp objects. Although exposures via biting and spitting have been reported and followed, none have led to an individual becoming infected.

In June 1996, the CDC released provisional recommendations regarding the efficacy of providing chemoprophylaxis following a significant bloody needlestick/sharp instrument injury. The postexposure prophylaxis (PEP) includes the use of two or three drugs. Each injury needs to be individually assessed in a timely fashion to determine if PEP is indicated.

Patients'/Clients' Risk of Acquiring HIV Infection in Healthcare Settings

Currently, the U.S. blood supply is generally considered safe from the risk of transmitting HIV. Not only is all donated blood tested for the presence of the HIV antibody, but donors are thoroughly screened to identify people who may be in the window period. Persons who think they may be at risk of being HIV-infected because of their sexual or needle-sharing history are discouraged from donating blood. Blood banks also discourage using blood donation as a way to discover one's HIV status. The current estimate is 2/1,000,000 units of transfused blood are infected.

The American Red Cross (ARC) began testing donated blood for the HIV antibody in 1985. It is estimated that, before testing, 4,770 individuals (4,476 adults and 294 children) became infected from blood transfusions; plus an additional 1,944 hemophiliac patients (1,775 adults and 169 children), from blood-clotting components. Currently, the ARC states that approximately 1/500,000 units/year may contain HIV (24 units/year). This is because of the window period, when an individual has acquired the virus but has not yet developed detectable antibodies. With the introduction of the p24 antigen test, which detects the presence of the virus, this estimate will drop to 1/700,000 units/year.

Testing programs are in place for donors of other body substances, such as semen, body organs, and body tissue. Since the donors of organs and body tissue have often died prior to donation, the ability to determine if the donor was in a window period of exposure to HIV is lost. Despite this problem, to date less than 20 cases have been reported as acquired by this route of infection.

Healthcare Worker-to-Patient Transmission

For an HIV-infected healthcare worker to pass the virus directly from themselves to a patient, the worker would literally have to bleed into a patient. This could occur only in specific situations, such as during a surgical procedure during which the infected individual cut or stuck themselves while inside a patient, thus allowing his or her blood to mingle with the patient's.

There is enough evidence to confirm six cases of HIV transmission from an HIV-infected Florida dentist to his patients. These individuals had no other confirmed exposures to HIV and few risk factors. DNA sequence analysis showed that the HIV strains had a high degree of similarity to that of the dentist and were distinct from the local control groups. The precise event(s) resulting in the transmissions are unknown. None of the patients had dental extractions or root canal therapies. Exposure to the dentist's blood cannot be ruled out, and the anesthetic needles and syringes may have been the transmission route.

The CDC has tested thousands of patients treated by HIV-infected healthcare workers. Although they have identified some HIV-infected patients, they have found no additional transmission links directly from infected healthcare workers. The risks for transmission from infected healthcare workers to patients is small and can be reduced with appropriate infection control precautions.

Patient-to-Patient Transmission

No cases of patient-to-patient HIV transmission have been documented in the United States. However, infection might occur if improperly cleaned, disinfected, or sterilized equipment or devices were used on several patients. It might also occur via the hands of personnel who did not wear, or properly change, gloves and/or did not wash their hands between patients. Both possibilities have been raised in the dental cases as well as a handful of other cases. It should be noted that, if transmission did occur via these routes, the HIV status of the healthcare worker would not necessarily be a factor. In other words, even an uninfected healthcare worker who does not practice proper infection control may be responsible for transmitting the disease from one patient to another.

In CMHCs, there is the possibility that patients will meet and subsequently engage in unprotected sexual intercourse or share needles. Patients might bite or spit on other patients or staff. However, there have been no reported HIV transmissions as a result of biting, spitting, or fighting. For transmission to occur as a result of these activities, the blood of one person would have to enter the body of another.

Preventing Workplace Exposure by Adhering to CDC Universal Precautions and OSHA Guidelines

The CDC's universal precautions guidelines, periodically updated, are intended to protect healthcare workers and patients from HIV, hepatitis B, hepatitis C, and other bloodborne pathogens. The precautions are directed to be used for all patients regardless of their age, diagnosis, or perceived behavioral risks.

A few weeks after the introduction of universal precautions, OSHA announced that they would become the enforcers of the guidelines because the CDC can issue recommendations but is not empowered to inspect for compliance. OSHA's own Bloodborne Pathogen Standard became effective March 6, 1992. All requirements had to be implemented by any agency or facility that provided any form of healthcare by July 6, 1992. It is important to note that OSHA's emphasis is on employee safety rather than on safety of patients, students, or volunteers. Only where there is an employer-employee relationship, in other words, a payment for service, is OSHA empowered to enforce standards. Agencies that must comply include those that offer mental health services, if the agency or facility performs any procedures where it could reasonably anticipate that a healthcare worker could sustain an occupational exposure such as a needlestick.

Procedures for Disposing of Sharp Instruments after Use

Healthcare workers may protect themselves from infection by a patient with HIV disease by following three basic kinds of precautions. First, respect sharp instruments such as needles and scalpels by using the following procedures.

1. Needles should not be recapped, bent, or broken. If they must be recapped, a recapping device, which holds the cap allowing only the hand holding the syringe and needle to be involved, or a one-handed scoop-up technique should be used.

2. Rigid, properly labeled, sharp instruments containers should be readily accessible to facilitate immediate disposal of uncapped needles or used sharp instruments (i.e., scalpels, tubes of blood, etc.). In CMHCs, this may mean bringing containers with you because it may not be feasible to have a container mounted in the room.

3. To avoid injury while injecting an agitated, uncooperative patient, you may

need the assistance of another person to hold or restrain the patient. Follow the same institutional guidelines for restraints that you would with any other patient.

Personal Precautions

Second, avoid direct contact with blood or body fluids of patients by using appropriate protective equipment. This precaution actually protects healthcare workers from patient transmission as well as patients from infected healthcare workers.

The use of personal protective equipment, gloves, gowns, goggles, etc., is determined by the procedure, or task, rather than the patient's diagnosis. Procedures that involve blood or other body substances dictate which protective barriers the worker should wear.

1. Gloves—should be worn when having direct contact with blood or any body substances (i.e., sputum, urine, feces, wound drainage).*

2. Gown or apron—should be worn if the worker's clothes may be soiled by blood or body substances.**

3. Mask and goggles (or face shield)—should be worn when close contact (within 3 feet) with respiratory secretions is anticipated (i.e., patient coughing, suctioning patient) or when there is a possibility of splashing or spraying into eyes or open mouth (i.e., with trauma patients or endoscopy, surgical procedures, irrigation of wounds).**

    * Equipment used for protection of patient and employee.
    ** Equipment used solely for protection of employee.

Hands should be vigorously washed after performing any procedure on any patient. The importance of proper handwashing cannot be emphasized enough for self-protection as well as protecting others from all types of pathogenic organisms, including HIV.

Healthcare workers who do direct, hands-on patient care should not perform certain procedures (surgery, dressing changes, etc.) when they have dermatitis or open cuts or lesions on their hands or forearms.

These major universal precautions protect healthcare workers from infection and, at the same time, protect patients from infection either from healthcare workers who are infected or from other patients. Appropriate wearing of personal protective equipment and handwashing after performing procedures is just standard, common sense infection control.

Handling Instruments and Equipment

Third, infection control requires properly cleaning any reusable devices, equipment, or instruments between patients. Healthcare workers should always either disinfect or sterilize equipment according to the following CDC guidelines regarding appropriate handling of instruments and/or equipment.

1. Equipment and devices that enter the patient's vascular (blood vessel) system, or other normally sterile areas of the body, should be sterilized before being used for each patient.

2. Equipment and devices that touch intact mucous membranes but do not penetrate the patient's body surfaces should be sterilized, when possible, or undergo high-level disinfection if they cannot be sterilized before being used for each patient.

3. Equipment and devices that do not touch the patient or that touch only intact skin of the patient need be cleaned only with a low-level disinfectant or as indicated by the manufacturer.

Once a CMHC determines the reusable equipment or instruments being used, it should develop appropriate procedures and establish mechanisms to ensure staff compliance.

Management of an Exposure

In the event that a worker sustains a percutaneous or mucocutaneous exposure, immediate first aid should be administered and the person should be taken to a facility that can provide appropriate medical care. The incident should be reported according to the policy of the CMHC.

Splashes to the eye, nose, mouth, or an open cut should be rinsed or washed, whichever is indicated. Punctures or sites of cuts created by the exposure should be cleansed with soap and water or an alcohol swipe.

Once the incident is reported to the appropriate medical personnel, an appropriate follow-up should be instituted. Follow-up may include injections of gamma globulin or hepatitis B vaccine and HIV blood testing of the injured person as well as the patient who is the source of the exposure. The use of chemoprophylaxis may be indicated based on the type of exposure and the source material involved. Prevailing recommendations should be consulted. Drugs used may include one or two antiretrovirals (e.g., AZT and 3TC) plus, in some instances, a protease inhibitor (e.g., indinavir or saquinavir).

If a CMHC offers or suggests the use of these drugs as part of postexposure

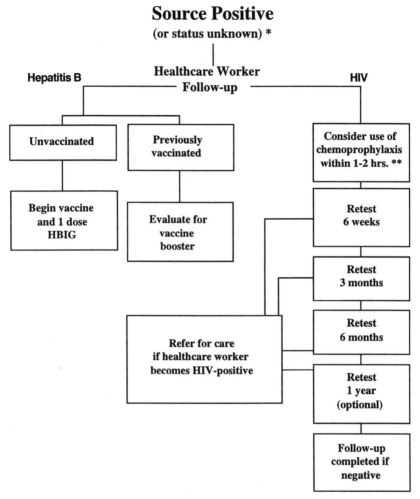

Source Positive

(or status unknown) *

Hepatitis B   **Healthcare Worker**   **HIV**
Follow-up

| Unvaccinated | Previously vaccinated | | Consider use of chemoprophylaxis within 1-2 hrs. ** |

| Begin vaccine and 1 dose HBIG | Evaluate for vaccine booster | | Retest 6 weeks |

Retest 3 months

| Refer for care if healthcare worker becomes HIV-positive | Retest 6 months |

Retest 1 year (optional)

Follow-up completed if negative

* If status of the source is unknown at the time of exposure, the Employee Health Office or designated clinician should facilitate getting the source and the health-care worker tested and institute follow-up on a case by case basis in accordance with state laws.

** It is imperitive to report any exposure immediately to facilitate appropriate evaluation to determine what, if any, chemoprophylaxis is indicated.

FIGURE 6.1 Management of an exposure.

management, the worker should receive appropriate counseling regarding potential side effects of the drugs. However, it is essential that the medication be initiated as soon after the exposure as possible if it is to have a beneficial effect. Individuals who provide postexposure follow-up should have current guidelines/recommendations available to ensure that the exposed worker is offered appropriate treatment. The HIV Division of the CDC is an excellent resource for this type of information.

In the rare event that a worker's baseline HIV test or follow-up test is found to be positive following an exposure, the worker should be referred for appropriate medical management of HIV disease. Community mental healthcare workers may be called upon to assist with counseling and emotional support for workers whose anxiety level may be quite high following an occupational exposure.

Postexposure counseling should minimally include:

1. A review of the specific HIV exposure and the risk of transmission

2. If the HIV exposure was determined to be significant, the importance of practicing safer sex until the serial testing is completed

3. The importance of completing the serial HIV testing as a way of reassuring the worker that no transmission occurred

4. In the rare event there was transmission, the importance of getting early medical care

Conclusion

The material covered here should reassure mental healthcare workers that the risk of acquiring HIV in a CMHC, while not zero, is certainly low. It is also low for patients. Obviously, it is prudent for clinicians and other workers to be conscious of what should be done to protect clients and staff from acquiring any disease in the healthcare setting.

Review Questions

1. How safe is the U.S. blood supply?
2. What is the primary mode of transmission from patient to healthcare worker?
3. What are the universal precautions for healthcare workers?
4. What should a healthcare worker do if exposed to HIV on the job?

5. What is the risk of occupationally acquiring hepatitis B compared with that of HIV?

References and Suggested Readings

American Health Consultants. AIDS alert: The monthly update for health professionals. Atlanta, GA: American Health Consultants, Inc., 3525 Piedmont Rd., Bldg. 6, Suite 400, Atlanta, GA 30305.

Baker, S.P., O'Neill, B., & Karpf, R.S. (1992). *The Injury Fact Book* (2nd ed.). New York: Oxford University Press.

Blank, S., Simonds, R.J., Weisfuse, I., Rudnick, J., Chiasson, M.A., & Thomas, P. (1994). Possible nosocomial transmission of HIV. *Lancet, 344,* 512–514.

Centers for Disease Control. (1987). Recommendations for prevention of HIV transmission in healthcare settings. *Morbidity and Mortality Weekly Report, 36,* Suppl. No. 25, 1–18S.

Centers for Disease Control. (1988). Update: Universal precautions for prevention of transmission of human immunodeficiency virus, hepatitis B virus, and other bloodborne pathogens in health-care settings. *Morbidity and Mortality Weekly Report, 37*(24), 377–382, 387–388.

Centers for Disease Control. (1991). Recommendations for preventing transmission of human immunodeficiency virus and hepatitis B virus to patients during exposure-prone invasive procedures. *Morbidity and Mortality Weekly Report, 40* (No. RR-8), 1–9.

Centers for Disease Control. (1993). Update: Investigations of patients who have been treated by HIV-infected health care workers—United States. *Morbidity and Mortality Weekly Report, 42*(17), 329–331, 337.

Centers for Disease Control and Prevention. (1995). Case-control study of HIV seroconversion in healthcare workers after percutaneous exposure to HIV-infected blood—France, United Kingdom, and United States, January 1988–August 1994. *Morbidity and Mortality Weekly Report, 44*(50), 929–933.

Centers for Disease Control and Prevention. (1996). Update: Provisional Public Health Service recommendations for chemoprophylaxis after occupational exposure to HIV. *Morbidity and Mortality Weekly Report, 45*(22), 468–472.

Charney, W., & Schirmer, J. (1990). *Essentials of Modern Hospital Safety.* Chelsea, MI: Lewis Publishers.

Gerberding, J.L. (1995). Management of occupational exposures to blood-borne viruses. *New England Journal of Medicine, 332*(7), 444–451.

Jagger, J., Hunt E.H., & Pearson, R.D. (1990). Estimated cost of needlestick injuries for six major needled devices. *Infection Control and Hospital Epidemiology, 11*(1), 584–588.

Jagger, J., Hunt, E.H., & Pearson, R.D. (1990). Sharp object injuries in the hospital: Causes and strategies for prevention. *American Journal of Infection Control, 18*(4), 227–231.

Jagger, J., Hunt, E.H., Brand-Elnaggar, J., & Pearson, R.D. (1988). Rates of needlestick injury caused by various devices in a university hospital. *New England Journal of Medicine, 319,* 284–288.

Occupational Safety and Health Administration. (1991). All about OSHA (rev.). Washington, D.C.: U.S. Department of Labor.

Occupational Safety and Health Administration. (1991). The standard. *Federal Register, 56*(235), 64175–64182.

Occupational Safety and Health Administration. (1989). OSHA inspections. Washington, DC: U.S. Deptartment of Labor.

Rowe, P.M., & Giuffre, M. (1991). Evaluating needlestick injuries in nursing personnel: Development of a questionnaire. *American Association of Occupational Health Nurses Journal 39,* 503–507.

Waller, J.A. (1985). *Injury Control: A Guide to the Causes and Prevention of Trauma.* Lexington, MA: Lexington Books.

Chapter 7

Medical Management

Robert P. Nelson, Jr., M.D.

Overview

This chapter seeks to familiarize community mental health center (CMHC) staff who are not physicians with the medical management of HIV and AIDS and with the multiple physical problems associated with HIV disease. Readers are introduced to diagnostic procedures, symptom management, common malignancies, and treatments. This information should help CMHC workers improve their ability to work with primary care physicians as well as better understand their clients' experience.

Learning Objectives

1. To understand the course of HIV disease.

2. To describe the approach to medical management of symptomatic patients.

3. To identify how HIV can affect individuals differently because of gender or age.

Outline

I. HIV Testing: Identification of HIV-Infected Persons

HIV Testing: Identification of HIV-Infected Persons

Human immunodeficiency virus (HIV) is a retrovirus that consists of proteins and genetic information in the form of ribonucleic acid (RNA). Structural proteins include an outer protein envelope, surface receptors for human cells called glyco-protein receptor (gp)120, and an inner core protein called p24.

The core surrounds the genetic material of the virus (RNA) and an enzyme called reverse transcriptase, which is necessary to transcribe the RNA to deoxyribonucleic acid (DNA). Subsequently, the DNA will direct the making of new viral proteins that will be cut to the correct lengths by a protease enzyme. Our current drugs against HIV attack the transcription process from RNA to DNA or inhibit the protease enzyme. The virus is inert and harmless until it touches an appropriate human cell; the glycoprotein receptor allows it to stick to the human cell and then enter it.

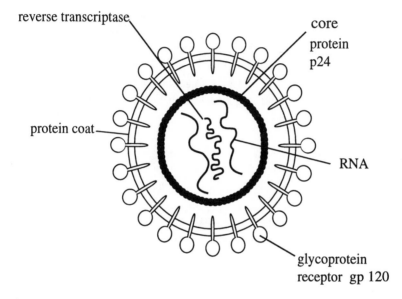

reverse transcriptase

core
protein
p24

protein coat

RNA

glycoprotein
receptor gp 120

FIGURE 7.1 Structure of the Human Immunodeficiency Virus

HIV infection causes antibodies to be produced by the infected person. Antibodies are protein molecules that are manufactured by immune cells and that circulate in the liquid part of the blood, the serum. Most infected persons become antibody-positive, or "seropositive," within six months of infection, and it is these antibodies that are detected when a person has an HIV test at a physician's office or health department. Most tests to determine infection, which now include the ELISA and Western blot, are tests for these antibodies.

A direct test for the virus itself measures a viral protein known as the p24 antigen, which is detectable in the serum of some HIV-infected persons. Viral DNA can also be detected by amplifying it in the laboratory through a technique known as the "PCR (polymerase chain reaction) test," which is particularly useful to diagnose HIV infection in newborns. Finally, RNA can be quantified in the plasma of infected persons and this is a measurement of how much virus is present in the circulation (viral load).

Management of Asymptomatic Patients

Natural History: Acute Infection

Following infection through exposure via mucous membranes, broken skin, or bloodstream invasion, the virus begins to replicate in one or more types of susceptible cells. Circulating CD4 lymphocytes, which are the "generals of the immunological army," and other immune cells known as monocytes are the most commonly infected cells. Within two to four weeks, infected persons often experience a flulike syndrome that includes fever, muscle aches and pains, lymph node enlargement, and sometimes a skin rash. This acute condition is rarely diagnosed, as these symptoms are nonspecific and are generally attributed to a benign viral illness such as influenza.

Asymptomatic Period

Following the acute flulike syndrome, adults with HIV may not feel symptoms for many years. This asymptomatic period is sometimes known as the incubation period or period of clinical latency. The median asymptomatic period for HIV-infected adults is 11 years. This means that, if 100 persons were infected all at the same time, 50 might still be asymptomatic 11 years later. Most infected individuals, therefore, are asymptomatic and not aware of their infection. Asymptomatic persons may, nonetheless, transmit the virus to others through blood transfusion, shared injection drug paraphernalia, unprotected sex and from mother to fetus.

Immune Deterioration

White Blood Cell Functions

- Neutrophils ("warriors") ingest and kill bacteria
- Lymphocytes ("generals")

  –CD4 helper cells: regulate immune responses

  –CD8 suppressor cells: kill virus-infected cells

The human immune system is designed to defend our tissues against bacteria, fungi, and viruses to which we are exposed. The main components of the immune system are white blood cells and antibodies. White blood cells include neutrophils (warrior cells), which ingest and kill bacteria, and lymphocytes (generals), which regulate immune responses and kill virus-infected cells. When a person has the common cold, for instance, virus-infected mucous membrane cells in the nose are identified and are killed by CD8 lymphocytes to prevent those cells from becoming factories to produce more viral particles. Another population of lymphocytes, called CD4 lymphocytes, recruits and directs other cells into the battle in a process called inflammation.

HIV creates a special problem because it infects the CD4 cells that direct the fight against infection. The body cannot compensate for the destruction caused by the billions of HIV particles produced each day. Large numbers of CD4 cells are lost each day and they are not fully replaced. Because the capacity of the immune system is large, years go by as the immune system gradually deteriorates. When the number of CD4 lymphocytes is insufficient to maintain good health, the patient becomes susceptible to a wide range of diseases, which take advantage of the weakened defenses of the body. These are known as opportunistic infections. Thus, HIV itself causes illness and also makes the person more susceptible to other diseases.

Infected persons who are not symptomatic may be evaluated by means of laboratory analyses of the blood. The number of CD4 lymphocytes can be counted. Normal numbers of CD4 lymphocytes in adults range from 450 to approximately 2000 per cubic millimeter of blood (cumm), with the majority having values between 800 and 1200. A patient who is infected with HIV experiences an average drop in this number of approximately 60 to 70 per year. Also, the number of viral particles in the blood can be estimated by the quantitative PCR test for RNA. These tests permit an estimate of the progression of the disease, even in a person without symptoms.

Informing Newly Diagnosed Patients

- Assess patient's level of knowledge.
- Assess patient's level of anxiety.
- Speak in language the patient understands.
- Give factual information with hope.
- Stress immediate goals.
- Identify support services.
- Initiate contact tracing.

A physician or other healthcare worker who is to inform a patient of his or her HIV status should assess the patient's level of knowledge and degree of anxiety and then present only what the patient can tolerate. Remember that patients who are hearing this information for the first time are usually emotionally overwhelmed and may not remember many of the details discussed. The information should be given in a form that the patient can understand. Repetition of the basic facts may be essential for comprehension.

The information presented must be factual. Medical information should include the HIV-related diagnostic medical terminology, as well as a lay description of the disease. The immediate aspects of the treatment plan should be stressed. The long duration of asymptomatic disease should be explained, as well as the rapidly expanding research. This provides a sense of hope. Positive aspects of patient care can be emphasized, including the ability to treat or prevent many of the secondary or opportunistic infections. The healthcare worker should be honest about the seriousness of HIV infection, but this honesty should be balanced with hope for the future.

During the discussion, the patient should also be told about available support. These include support groups, social service agencies, religious organizations, family, and friends. Many questions will surface (e.g., "Should I continue to work?" "What is my prognosis?" "Will I infect my partner?"). These questions need to be answered both simply and directly. Though often an uncomfortable topic, the issue of transmission to sexual partners should be addressed and public health directed contact tracing may be initiated. Partners should be offered testing options. Physicians should be familiar with the requirements for contact tracing in their state. These requirements should be explained to the patient so that the appropriate action can be taken with the patient's knowledge.

Early Signs and Symptoms

- Weight loss
- Skin sores
- Diarrhea
- Sore throat
- Mouth ulcers
- Persistent cough
- Lymph node enlargement

- Fever
- Weakness
- Rash
- Night sweats
- Purple spots on skin
- Facial skin rash
- Poor memory and confusion

The mental healthcare worker may hear of physical complaints that need to be referred to the physician. These include fatigue, unexplained fevers, unintentional weight loss, weakness, nonhealing cold sores (herpes simplex infections), chronic skin conditions, oral or vaginal candidiasis (yeast infection), and unexplained diarrhea. Presence of night sweats sufficient to drench pajamas or bedding are characteristic symptoms of HIV infection.

Examination

The physician will examine the patient for physical findings, which include weight loss, elevated temperature, changes in the appearance of the eye, oral candidiasis, hairy leukoplakia, and herpes simplex, or mouth ulcers. Listening to the chest may reveal crackles or wheezing in patients who have early *Pneumocystis* pneumonia. The skin is sometimes abnormal in patients with HIV. For example, some patients have dry, flaking skin; others may have unusually severe psoriasis or reddish or reddish brown tumors of the skin called Kaposi's sarcoma. The perianal region is examined for signs of rash or ulcers. Patients with HIV infection often have swelling in the lymph nodes and these may be found in the neck area, under the arms, and in the groin. Neurological examination may reveal weakness or sensory loss on either side of the body. Change in mental status may be a subtle finding early in the course of the HIV infection.

Laboratory Testing
1. Blood chemistry profile
2. Blood count
3. VDRL (syphilis) test
4. Hepatitis B profile test
5. Tuberculin skin test
6. CD4 lymphocyte count
7. PCR test for viral RNA

Patients who are diagnosed as HIV-infected should have laboratory tests to rule out the presence of other diseases and to establish baselines, which may be compared to future evaluations. These tests include the following:

1. A blood chemistry profile should be conducted to establish liver and kidney function. Enzymes spill into the circulation when liver cells are damaged and there are chemicals that increase in the bloodstream when the kidneys are not working normally.

2. A complete blood count will detect abnormalities of the red blood cells and white blood cells (which fight infection). The platelet count measures the cell fragments which aid in blood clotting.

3. A screening test for syphilis (VDRL or RPR) will be done. If this is positive, another test called an FTA (or MHPT) should be done to confirm that syphilis is present so that treatment may be initiated.

4. A hepatitis B profile test should be obtained so that persons with active

infection can be identified. Persons without hepatitis B immunity should be immunized.

5. A tuberculin skin test should be done to establish whether the patient has been infected with tuberculosis (TB). Even if the infection is not active, it may require treatment to prevent it from becoming active.

6. CD4 lymphocytes should be measured to provide an estimate of how far the disease has progressed.

7. The number of viral particles in the blood can be measured with the quantitative RNA PCR test. This test is used for staging and monitoring levels that predict disease progression. This test may also indicate the effectiveness of antiretroviral (anti-HIV) medications; the response to antiretroviral therapy is rapid—usually within three to four weeks.

The most commonly performed test, used to determine when a patient should be treated, is the CD4 lymphocyte count. The normal range for adults is 800–1200 per cumm of blood. Individuals with CD4 counts of less than 200 are at risk for *Pneumocystis* pneumonia, which requires prophylactic treatment.

HIV illness is understood as a continuum from asymptomatic to symptomatic disease, the course of which is characterized by progressive depletion of CD4 lymphocyte numbers and functioning. There has been increasing emphasis placed on the use of antiretroviral therapy during the asymptomatic period, although there are still questions regarding the best agent(s) to use. This is an area of intensive research. The quantitative RNA (viral load) is emerging as an important guide for starting or changing antiretroviral therapy.

It is important to realize that the CD4 lymphocyte count may fluctuate with time of day, concurrent viral infections, psychological depression, or other unknown factors, so the interpretation of the count should be made with caution. Repeated measurements, that is, every three to six months, are recommended so that antiretroviral therapy will not be initiated because of an aberrantly low value or therapy will not be withheld because of an aberrantly high value.

In 1987, it was demonstrated that antiretroviral therapy with zidovudine (AZT) was successful in prolonging life and reducing opportunistic infection. Since then, other medications that also inhibit the viral enzyme reverse transcriptase have been made available, including didanosine (ddI), zalcitabine (ddC), stavudine (D4T), lamivudine (3TC), nevirapine (Viramune), and delavirdine. Three of these compounds, AZT, ddI, and 3TC are approved for use in children. A new class of drugs, called protease inhibitors provides four additional antiretroviral agents (saquinavir, ritonavir, nelfinavir, and indinavir), which are potent inhibitors of viral replication.

AZT and ddI prolong survival, increase CD4 counts, delay progression to AIDS, improve HIV-associated dementia, improve platelet counts in HIV-associated thrombocytopenia (low platelet count), and decrease viral load (amount of viral RNA in the blood). The timely approval of nevirapine and the protease inhibitors in 1995–97 and the knowledge that rapid viral replication occurs throughout the course of HIV have led to renewed interest and optimism in antiretroviral therapy.

Multiple studies now demonstrate that AZT monotherapy is no longer the treatment of choice except for HIV-infected pregnant women. "Triple" therapy, which is treatment with three antiretroviral medications, is currently thought of as the most aggressive and potent approach and is advocated for most patients with CD4 counts less than $200/mm^3$. There are also advocates for combination therapy for people with earlier stage diseases, although the effectiveness in this treatment is not known at this time.

Antiretroviral therapeutic agents have toxicities and drug interactions that complicate their use. Protease inhibitor compounds (indinavir, ritonavir, nelfinavir, and saquinavir) alter the cytochrome P-450 enzyme system, which affects the metabolism of many drugs. These interactions are especially important for patients treated with psychotropic medications. Ritonavir, for instance, leads to a moderate increase in tricyclic antidepressant blood levels. It is the goal of ongoing clinical trials to ascertain the best agent or combination of agents to prolong life, delay disease progression, and improve the quality of life.

Management of Symptomatic Patients

Evaluation and Differential Diagnosis of Constitutional Symptoms

Constitutional signs and symptoms are nonspecific in nature. These include fever, night sweats, weight loss, and chronic diarrhea. The reason these are nonspecific is that they may be caused by many other illnesses besides HIV. Patients may start to develop symptoms of illness when the CD4 lymphocyte number drops below 350 per cumm of blood. Most patients experience symptoms when lymphocyte counts are below 200. The goal is to identify the cause of the symptoms and to provide specific treatment. Fatigue is one of the most common symptoms associated with HIV infection. This fatigue is often profound and requires the patient to take naps, especially in the late afternoon. Fatigue may also be a sign of conditions that can accompany HIV infection, such as anemia or opportunistic infection. A thorough history, physical examination, and laboratory tests should be done to evaluate new symptoms in the HIV-infected patient.

Organ System Evaluation

Multiple organ systems can be affected by HIV disease. Primary care physicians must treat or coordinate the treatment of diseases of all of these systems. This multiple organ system effect makes treatment both complex and costly. Common problems that HIV patients may experience include:

Neuropsychiatric Problems

- HIV encephalopathy
- Depressive syndrome
- Medication complications
- Opportunistic infection of the nervous system
- Central nervous system malignancy

Neuropsychiatric symptoms include mental status abnormalities such as forgetfulness, confusion, mood changes, and dementia. These may be the first symptoms experienced by up to 30 percent of the patients with HIV infection. Neurological symptoms occur in 65 percent of the patients at some time during the course of their illness, and at autopsy 95 percent of the patients are found to have significant neurological involvement. Physicians can refer patients for neuropsychological testing, which may help to distinguish between an organic dementia and depression, both of which may accompany HIV infection. Medications may also cause nervous system dysfunction, including peripheral neuropathy. Opportunistic infections of the central nervous system include toxoplasmosis caused by a parasite and cryptococcal meningitis caused by a fungus. Evaluation of central nervous system symptoms often includes radiographic imaging, such as computerized tomography (CT) or magnetic resonance imaging (MRI) of the head. Cancers of the brain in HIV-infected patients are mostly lymph system cancers called lymphomas. Patients sometimes undergo lumbar punctures (spinal taps) for spinal fluid analysis in an effort to identify the cause of the neurological symptoms.

Dermatologic Problems

- Nonspecific inflammation
- HIV infection of skin
- Herpes zoster
- Herpes simplex

- Fungal infection
- Impetigo
- Excessive reaction to mosquito bites

The skin is one of the most commonly affected organs in HIV disease. Some skin cells are actually infected by the virus. Other infections include herpes zoster, herpes simplex, fungal infections, and impetigo caused by bacteria. Patients will often have excessive reactions to mosquito bites and may have an actual breakdown of the skin with scabbing. Herpes simplex, which causes cold sores that last three to five days in persons who are not HIV-infected, may cause festering scabbed lesions that may last two to three weeks in persons with HIV. Herpes zoster, which is the varicella or chicken pox virus, causes shingles involving small areas of skin in healthy people; HIV-infected people usually have multiple areas with more extensive involvement. This is frequently a sign of advanced HIV disease.

Ophthalmologic Problems

- Cytomegalovirus (CMV)
- Toxoplasmosis

The most common cause of visual problems in HIV-infected persons is retinitis or inflammation of the retina caused by CMV. It occurs almost exclusively in those with CD4 lymphocyte counts of less than 100 per cumm. Up to 20 percent of the patients with HIV may initially present with the symptom of blurred vision related to CMV retinitis. For this reason, regular ophthalmological examinations are recommended for patients with HIV infection and CD4 counts below 150. Toxoplasmosis may also cause blindness in patients with HIV infection, but this is much less common.

Ear, Nose, and Throat Problems

- Sinusitis

Three of the most common complaints of patients with HIV infection are nasal congestion, runny nose, and cough. There is high incidence of sinusitis (infection of the sinuses). These individuals may need a longer duration of antibiotic treatment than someone who is not HIV-infected, and recurrences of sinus infection are common.

Pulmonary Problems

- *Pneumocystis* pneumonia
- Bacterial pneumonias
- Tuberculosis

Over half of HIV-infected patients eventually present with symptoms of lower respiratory tract infection (pneumonia). The most common cause of pneumonia is an opportunistic organism known as *Pneumocystis carinii*. Rather than waiting to treat this condition after the individual becomes ill, prophylaxis (administration of anti-*Pneumocystis* therapy before the occurrence of active infection) is now used to prevent this problem. It is important that infected individuals regularly take trimethoprim-sulfamethoxazole (Bactrim/Septra) or an alternative when the CD4 count drops below 200 per cumm. Bacterial pneumonias may also occur. Recently, there has been a significant increase in the number of cases of TB. All patients with HIV infection must be evaluated for TB infection and treated and followed closely if TB infection is present.

Cardiovascular Problems

- Congestive heart failure

The heart is noticeably spared in the course of most HIV infections. Some patients eventually develop congestive heart failure, probably owing to disease of the heart muscle caused by direct HIV infection. Congestive heart failure may also occur in children.

Gastrointestinal Problems

- Oral candidiasis (thrush)
- Herpes simplex
- Mouth ulcers (canker sores)
- Diarrhea

Oral lesions are common in HIV-infected persons. Aphthous ulcers (canker sores) are large painful ulcers of the oral cavity. Treatment is not often effective. Candidiasis, a fungal disease that causes vaginitis in many women, rarely occurs in the mouths of people without HIV infection, but is common in persons with HIV infection. While easily treated, it may require prolonged therapy. Herpes simplex causes cold sores of the oral cavity which are common and treatable. Periodontal disease of a particularly aggressive nature also occurs. Diarrhea is one of the most common symptoms associated with HIV infection and may be caused by HIV or be secondary to bacterial, parasite, fungal, mycobacterial, or viral organisms. It is frequently a debilitating symptom and is difficult to treat.

Muscle and Joint Problems

- HIV arthropathy
- Chlamydia infections
- Myositis (HIV-related or AZT-related)

Some patients with HIV infection develop joint and muscle aches and pains. These may be related to HIV itself or be secondary to an immune response or to an infection such as chlamydia. There is a clinical syndrome characterized by the weakness of large muscles and associated with extreme fatigue. Also, AZT may cause a rare form of inflammation of the muscles (myositis).

Hormonal Problems

- Low testosterone

Although the adrenal gland and pituitary function may be altered secondary to HIV or opportunistic disease, the most common endocrine abnormality in HIV is a low serum testosterone level. There is some correlation between a low serum testosterone level, weight loss, and low lymphocyte counts in males. Testosterone should, therefore, be measured in male patients who experience weight loss. Replacement testosterone therapy may be helpful.

Hematologic Problems

- Chronic anemia

Anemia occurs frequently in symptomatic HIV patients. Causes of anemia include the so-called anemia of chronic disease, AZT therapy, and systemic infections. Anemia may be treated with blood transfusions, alteration in dosage or type of antiretroviral medication, or provision of growth factors that stimulate red blood cell production.

Wasting Syndrome

Wasting syndrome is a malnourished state in which people lose weight despite adequate nutritional intake. It may occur even in carefully managed patients and may be related to viral replication, secondary infection (especially atypical mycobacteria), malnutrition, the development of a malignancy, or to some combination of factors.

Malignant Complications of HIV

When the immune system is suppressed, it may not adequately protect the body against the growth of cancers. The two most common cancers that occur in HIV-infected persons are lymphomas and Kaposi's sarcoma. They may cause severe complications.

Lymphoma

- Aggressive and fast-growing lymphoma
- Rapid weight loss and fatigue
- Investigation of dominant lymph nodes
- Treated with chemotherapy or radiation palliation and pain control

Lymphomas that develop in HIV-infected persons are particularly aggressive and fast-growing. They may cause symptoms of rapid weight loss, fevers, night sweats, and fatigue. The occurrence of a swollen lymph node in the neck, under the arm, or in the groin may be caused by infection or may indicate the presence of lymphoma. It should be examined by a physician and a diagnostic biopsy may be appropriate. Lymphomas are generally treated with aggressive chemotherapy if the person's physical condition can tolerate such therapy.

Kaposi's Sarcoma

- Common in homosexual/bisexual males
- Rare in women and children
- Affects skin and sometimes lymph nodes and organs
- Multiple treatments available

Kaposi's sarcoma is a growth of blood vessels in the skin and/or on various organs inside the body. It occurs in up to 30 percent of homosexual males with HIV infection, but infrequently in children and women with HIV infection. Kaposi's sarcoma may affect any portion of the skin or oral cavity and usually appears as pink to red-brown spots, nodules, or tumors. Multiple treatments are available to help people with Kaposi's sarcoma. Rigorous diagnosis with appropriate treatment is indicated.

HIV Infection in Women

- 15% of reported cases
- Similar symptoms as those in males, plus genitourinary problems, such as venereal warts and cervical cancer
- Needs gynecological examination and PAP smear at least every six months

Fifteen percent of the cases of HIV infection in the United States occur in women, and the proportion of new cases of AIDS diagnosed in women is increasing. HIV infection in women may be manifested by all of the symptoms discussed, with the addition of genitourinary problems such as venereal warts and cervical cancer. For this reason, women require gynecological examinations at least every six months. (See Chapter 15, "Women and HIV.")

Pediatric AIDS

Pediatric patients are defined by the Centers for Disease Control and Prevention as those under age 13. Pediatric AIDS cases include children who became infected through blood transfusion or from being born to an HIV-infected mother. The incidence of transmission of HIV to infants from an infected mother is approximately 15 to 30 percent without antiretroviral intervention. This means that most infants born to seropositive mothers, although temporarily antibody positive (because they receive the antibodies from the mother even if they do not receive the virus) are actually not infected. Transmission to a fetus depends on multiple factors, the most important of which is whether an antiretroviral therapy program was used during pregnancy and labor and postnatally. Research has demonstrated that AZT, when given to previously untreated mothers and their newborn offspring, can reduce the transmission rate by 67 percent. This is one of the main reasons why HIV tests for pregnant women should be universally provided.

Children with HIV infection suffer from opportunistic infections similar to adults. A relatively high frequency of bacterial pneumonias and bloodstream infections is unique to children. Recurrent sinusitis and ear infections are troublesome problems. Oral polio vaccination (a live virus vaccine) should not be given to infants at risk for HIV because there is the theoretical risk of the vaccine actually causing polio in a severely immunodeficient child. Fortunately, there is a suitable intramuscular alternative available (a killed virus vaccine).

HIV in Elderly Persons

The diagnosis of HIV in elderly persons is complicated by the perception of many healthcare providers that risk activities are not present in this population. Fewer than half of elderly individuals have had previous blood transfusions as a sole risk factor for HIV infection. Research has shown that about 10 percent of elderly Americans have at least one risk factor. Sexual or drug-associated risk behaviors account for most infections in this population. A very small proportion of the elderly use condoms during sex or have undergone HIV testing.

HIV infection in the elderly is usually not considered by clinicians until late in the course of infection, because many fail to recognize this possibility. Encephalopathy and other cognitive disorders may be the presenting symptoms, and because dementia is common in the elderly, the clinician must have a high index of suspicion to diagnose HIV in a timely fashion. In this population, it is often difficult to determine whether dementia is caused by HIV infection.

Heart conditions, hypertension, diabetes, depression, and other chronic disorders may complicate the medical management of HIV disease in the elderly. Symptoms of HIV and its infectious complications may mimic those that occur secondary to these disorders, and medication interactions may be complex and clinically important. Additional management complications occur because the progression of HIV to AIDS and death is accelerated in elderly persons as compared to that in younger populations.

Treatment for Persons with HIV

Five Mainstays of Treatment

1. Antiretroviral therapy
2. Prophylaxis of opportunistic infections
3. Treatment of infectious diseases (and/or malignancies)
4. Nutritional support
5. Psychosocial assessment and support

The five mainstays of treatment for patients with symptomatic HIV illness include the provision of optimal antiretroviral therapy, prophylaxis of opportunistic infections, specific treatment for secondary infectious diseases (and/or malignancies), provision of appropriate nutritional support, and psychosocial assessment and support.

The current antiretroviral therapies include AZT, ddI, ddC, D4T 3TC, nevirapine, and delavirdine, all of which interfere with the reverse transcriptase enzyme. These may be used alone or in combination. Recently approved protease enzyme inhibitors include saquinavir, ritonavir, indinavir, and Nelfinavir. Drugs are available that may prevent or treat herpes simplex, candidiasis, toxoplasmosis, *Pneumocystis* pneumonia, atypical tuberculosis, and CMV.

Adequate nutrition, sufficient rest, and exercise are necessary to resist infections and to maintain a sense of well-being. Psychosocial support is essential for the patient's emotional stability. Each of these five areas is equally important in the overall care of the HIV-infected individual.

Care Systems

- Outpatient
- Inpatient
- Home healthcare
- Hospice
- Clinical trials

Most of the care of the HIV-infected person is provided in an outpatient setting. Because of the ability to predict clinical illness and to provide prophylaxis, patients may be treated indefinitely as outpatients. Hospitalization is necessary for seriously ill patients or for those who require surgical procedures. The provision of home healthcare services has reduced the length of hospital stays. Experienced groups of home healthcare nurses and pharmacists may prepare infusions, obtain laboratory testing, and monitor response to treatment.

As the patient nears the terminal stage of illness, hospice services may be appropriate. Patients require adequate analgesia for pain. Decisions regarding extreme measures to prolong life, such as mechanical ventilation, should be discussed while the patient is still lucid, and the care plan should be communicated to the hospice workers.

All patients with HIV are candidates for participation in clinical trials. Clinical trials provide experimental medications to individuals to determine the effectiveness of the medication in treating HIV infection. There is a nationwide network of clinical trial centers known as the AIDS Clinical Trial Group.

Conclusion

HIV causes a gradual loss of immune function, which results in a gradual increase in susceptibility to opportunistic infections. Over a period of years most infected persons develop nonspecific signs and symptoms of HIV illness and, later, experience opportunistic infections and/or wasting syndrome. Malignancies occur with greatly increased frequency in HIV-infected persons.

Early diagnosis and therapy is emphasized as the rational approach to proper medical management. Therapies are currently available which directly inhibit HIV replication and prevent or treat troublesome secondary infections. Nutritional and psychosocial supportive care are important adjuncts to the medical management of HIV disease. There must be effective communication between the patient, mental health professional, physician, and other members of the healthcare team to enhance the patient's quality of life and maximize life expectancy.

Review Questions

1. What do the most commonly used tests for HIV in adults actually measure?
2. Which cell is the major target for HIV?
3. Name and describe three constitutional signs/symptoms of HIV illness.
4. What is the most frequent cause of pneumonia in HIV-infected adults?

References and Suggested Readings

Broder, S., Merigan, T.C., & Bolognesi, D. (Eds.) (1994). *Textbook of AIDS Medicine*. Baltimore: Williams & Wilkins.

Centers for Disease Control. (1995). First 500,000 AIDS cases—United States, 1995. *Morbidity and Mortality Weekly Report, 44,* 849–853.

Collier, A.C., Coombs, R.W., Schoenfeld D.A., Bassett, R.L., Timpone, J.T., Baruch, A., Jones, M., Facey, K., Whitacre, C., McAuliffe, V.J., Friedman, H.M., Merigan, T.C., Reichman, R.C., Hooper, C., & Corey, L. (1996). Treatment of human immunodeficiency virus infection with saquinavir, zidovudine and zalcitabine. *New England Journal of Medicine, 334,* 1011–1017.

Conner, E.M., Sperling, R.S., Gelber, R., Kiselev, P., Scott, G., O'Sullivan, M.J., VanDyke, R., Bey, M., Shearer, W., & Jacobson, R.L. (1994). Reduction of maternal-infant transmission of human immunodeficiency virus Type 1 with zidovudine treatment. *New England Journal of Medicine, 331,* 1173–1180.

Danner, S.A., Carr, A., Leonard, J.M., Lehman, L.M., Gudiol, F., Gonzales, J., Raventos, A., Rubio, R., Bouza, E., & Pintado, V. (1995). A short-term study of the safety, pharmacokinetics and efficacy of vitoravir, an inhibitor of HIV-1 protease. *New England Journal of Medicine, 33,* 1528–1533.

Fischl, M.A., Richman, D.D., Grieco, M.H., Gottlieb, M.S., Volberding, P.A., Laskin, O.L., Leedom, J.M., Groopman, J.E., Mildvan, D., Schooley, R.T., Jackson, G.G., Durack, D.T., & King, D. (1987). The efficacy of azidothymidine (AZT) in the treatment of patients with AIDS and AIDS-related complex. A double-blind, placebo-controlled trial. *New England Journal of Medicine, 317,* 185–191.

Hirsch, M.S., & D'Aquila, R.T. (1993). Therapy for human immunodeficiency virus infection. *New England Journal of Medicine, 328,* 1686–1695.

Ho, D.D., Neumann, A.U., Perelson, A.S., Chen, W., Leonard, J.M., & Markowitz, M. (1995). Rapid turnover of plasma virions and CD4 lymphocytes in HIV-1 infection. *Nature 373,* 123–126.

Mellors, J.W., Kingsley, L.A., Rinaldo, C.R., Todd, J.A., Hoo, B.S., Kokka, R.P., & Gupta, P. (1995). Quantitation of HIV-1 RNA in plasma predicts outcome after seroconversion. *Annals of Internal Medicine, 122,* 573–579.

Rabbat, A.S., Ong, K.R., & Glatt, A.E. (1996). Pain—a frequently forgotten finding in HIV infection. *AIDS Reader, Jan/Feb,* 6–12.

USPHS/IDSA guidelines for the prevention of opportunistic infections in persons infected with human immunodeficiency virus: A summary. (1996). *Annals of Internal Medicine, 124,* 349–360.

Chapter 8

Working with Primary Care Physicians

Charles F. Clark, M.D., M.P.H.

Overview

This chapter prepares community mental health center (CMHC) staff to create alliances with primary care physicians to link clients with HIV disease to appropriate healthcare. It includes a review of common problems in traditional medical settings that interfere with HIV patient care. Suggestions for locating primary care physicians are included, as are strategies for forging alliances with them. The importance of a communitywide HIV working group is stressed.

Learning Objectives

1. To identify three problems that impede the interest or ability of primary care physicians to care for patients with HIV disease.

2. To suggest three ways to encourage primary care physicians to participate in the care of HIV/AIDS patients.

3. To understand the importance of community agencies participating in an HIV/AIDS working group.

Outline

    I. Problems for Primary Care Physicians Providing HIV/AIDS Patient Care

      A. Problems in education and training

      B. Behavior physicians find difficult to tolerate

    II. Economic and Political Issues That Affect Treatment of HIV-Positive Patients

      A. Problems of availability and cost

        1. HIV/AIDS medical care is expensive

        2. Specialized care

        3. Experimental or extremely expensive drugs

      B. AIDS care outside the medical model

    III. Locating Appropriate Primary Care Physicians for HIV/AIDS Patients

    IV. Forging Alliances with Primary Care Providers

    V. Developing a Community HIV/AIDS Working Group to Coordinate and Solicit Care

Problems for Primary Care Physicians Providing HIV/AIDS Patient Care

The provision of medical care for HIV/AIDS patients has been a contentious issue within the American medical establishment as well as within American society. The following list identifies some of the problems in the education and training of primary care physicians regarding HIV/AIDS.

Problems in Education and Training

- Physicians share beliefs and prejudices common to other members of society.
- Many physicians have no training in HIV/AIDS.
- Many physicians have no experience with HIV/AIDS.
- Only physicians in practice less than ten years learned about AIDS in medical school.

Physicians, as members of our society, have the same beliefs and prejudices about AIDS as other people. Although we want to believe that no physician will have prejudices about patients, that is simply unrealistic.

HIV/AIDS is a new disease and most physicians have had little training in the care of HIV/AIDS patients unless they began practicing after 1988. Unless a physician goes on to practice in a setting that specializes in serving AIDS patients, she or he may not have the opportunity to learn about new developments in AIDS treatment or the realities of patient care. A multiyear educational effort by the Public Health Service to educate physicians about AIDS and to encourage them to care for persons with AIDS is currently under way.

Physicians have expectations of their patients' behavior that are not always realistic and that are troublesome to many AIDS patients. The following list includes behavior that is difficult for many physicians to tolerate.

Behavior Physicians Find Difficult to Tolerate

- Not keeping appointments
- Not being on time
- Not having laboratory tests done
- Not taking medications as prescribed
- Taking nonprescribed medications
- Not behaving as grateful patients

Economic and Political Issues That Affect Treatment of HIV-Positive Patients

The economic and political realities of the American medical system discourage the primary care physician from caring for AIDS patients or, depending on one's point of view, provide an excuse for the physician to avoid providing care.

Problems of Availability and Cost

- High cost of HIV/AIDS medical care
  - Need to be wealthy or have excellent medical insurance
  - Most patients ending up on Medicaid with poor reimbursement of physician, pharmacist, and laboratory

- Availability and cost of specialized care

    –CD4 (T-cell) counts

    –CT and MRI scans

- Availability of experimental drugs or extremely expensive drugs

    –Need to be on an experimental protocol

    –Elaborate paperwork required to access expensive drugs

This list illustrates some of the problems for physicians in caring for AIDS patients. It is difficult to provide adequate care because AIDS is an expensive disease to treat. It is expensive in physician and nurse time, in the cost of medications, and in the cost of the laboratory tests necessary to evaluate the progress of the disease. Although many persons have adequate medical insurance through their employment, the insurance is often lost when they become too ill to work. This forces patients into federal and state medical assistance programs that are widely acknowledged to be inadequate in physician, laboratory, hospital, and medication reimbursement. Few persons are wealthy enough to pay for their own AIDS care. Additionally, the disease disproportionately affects the poor and disadvantaged members of society.

Several of the tests needed to follow the progress of the disease, such as CD4 (T-cell) counts and CT and MRI scans, are available only in large medical centers. Many of the medications necessary to treat the disease and its complications are experimental and available only if the physician and his or her patients are part of a research program protocol. In addition, most of the medications are expensive, and elaborate applications must be completed to obtain them with public funds.

For a number of political, social, and economic reasons, the treatment of AIDS as a disease has occurred outside of the traditional medical model.

AIDS Care Outside the Medical Model

- AIDS care was forced on a reluctant medical system.
- Patients and activists developed treatment approaches.
- AIDS patients and activists forced the availability of drugs.
- Only young physicians "grew up" with AIDS.
- Older physicians are just learning how to treat AIDS.
- AIDS patients expect more control over their treatment:

–Tell the doctor what to give them;

–Use underground drugs (the physician doesn't approve or doesn't want to know).

AIDS care was forced upon a reluctant medical system. In response to government and medical establishment foot-dragging, individuals infected with the virus, their friends, and allies were instrumental in developing models of care outside of the traditional medical system. Medications became available only because of direct patient political action or even overt drug smuggling.

The political and social climate and the overt discrimination affecting HIV-infected persons have served to make the AIDS patient a much more active participant in decisions about his or her own medical care than the usual patient. While this is good in many ways, it places an added burden on the primary physician who must not only treat a strange new disease, but must do so in a patient/physician relationship that is unfamiliar. AIDS patients are likely to tell a doctor what to prescribe or how they expect to be treated professionally. They are often using non-FDA-approved drugs, which the physician does not sanction, is unfamiliar with, or does not want to know about. Only young physicians who completed training after AIDS became widespread are accustomed to working with AIDS patients in this new model. Older physicians are, only now, learning how to treat AIDS and work with HIV-infected persons.

Locating Appropriate Primary Care Physicians for HIV/AIDS Patients

There are some positive aspects of physician training that can be relied upon to facilitate securing sensitive care for HIV-infected persons. Physicians' education and training promote medical ideals of charitable patient care, social tolerance, and community service. While physicians, like many in their local communities, may be prejudiced against male homosexuals and injecting drug users, they feel obligated to provide medical care to persons who are ill as a humanitarian community service. Therefore, any physician may be approached about providing care for an AIDS patient with a reasonable expectation that the physician will either provide the care or assist in locating a source of care.

Particularly in rural areas, it may be difficult to find a public health clinic or a physician who is already known to be willing to care for AIDS patients. Community mental healthcare workers may need to help the patient find a willing physician. They may appeal to physicians' dedication to community service, humanitarian ideals, and reputation for tolerance. Most people, if appealed to by attributing the most positive assumptions, will attempt to live up to expectations.

The younger the physician, the more likely she or he is to be knowledgeable about the care of AIDS patients. General practitioners, pediatricians, and internists are the most appropriate primary care physicians for AIDS patients. Those whose practices are developing may have the extra time to learn about AIDS and care for these new patients. Those with full, busy practices have the income that will permit them to care for some nonpaying or partially paying patients. The CMHC worker can ask the physician directly if he or she is able and willing to care for the person with AIDS.

Where there are no physicians with experience in caring for AIDS patients, it is important to choose a physician, and physician's staff, with whom the CMHC worker feels comfortable because, together, they will be learning to care for AIDS patients. The physician must be willing to learn new skills and new ways of relating to patients. While young physicians may be thought to be more adaptable, many older physicians have seen and heard the worst that life can offer and have an understanding of human behavior that would make them ideal AIDS caregivers.

Forging Alliances with Primary Care Physicians

Caring for patients with HIV infection, particularly as it progresses to AIDS, is frustrating and frequently discouraging work. Health and mental healthcare providers are caring for young and middle-aged people in the productive years of their lives who are dying of a preventable infectious disease. Despite the frequent news of scientific breakthroughs, the long-term survival experience of these patients is discouraging.

Forging an Alliance with Primary Care Physicians

- Acknowledge the frustration of caring for patients dying of a preventable infectious disease.
- Share knowledge about the patient's need for autonomy expressed through the use of alternative therapies.
- Share information about underground drugs.
- Provide neuropsychiatric and psychosocial consultation for physicians.
- Tell the physician about interesting educational opportunities.
- Ask the physician to teach your staff about AIDS.

The preceeding list identifies some of the ways in which CMHC staff and physicians may interact in treating HIV-infected persons. It is essential that staff and the physician support and educate one another during the effort to provide AIDS care. Community mental health center clinicians can explain to the physician the psychological need or rationale for the patient participating in alternative therapies. The CMHC may locate courses or educational opportunities about AIDS that the physician might find useful. Such training should not be limited solely to medical treatments, but may include discussions about psychological issues, nutritional needs, epidemiology, and other relevant subjects.

Community mental health center staff may have the opportunity to observe symptoms, such as difficulty comprehending medical instructions, erratic behavior, and poor compliance with treatment regimens that indicate the onset of neuropsychiatric complications in clients who are HIV-positive. The treating physician may initially be puzzled or even angered by this behavior, which may be the outward manifestation of early AIDS dementia or secondary infections of the brain. The CMHC staff can alert a physician to these possibilities since the client may require specialized tests and changes in the treatment plan.

Clinicians may provide psychosocial consultation to physicians and monitor clients' attitudes, behavior, and compliance with medical treatment. Simultaneously, CMHC counselors may develop an understanding of the attitudes and treatment style of physicians and medical staffs. They may be in a position to help either clients or physicians to modify behavior and treatment regimens so that the client receives maximum benefit from the available medical resources. Staff have an opportunity to share with physicians a global view of the treatment process that includes the social, psychological, and economic, as well as medical, aspects of treatment. This perspective is an asset that physicians can appreciate and use when developing treatment plans.

Physicians like to teach. Encourage rapport by asking the physician to teach CMHC staff about AIDS medical care, not the esoteric details of drug treatment, but practical knowledge such as how to recognize signs of deterioration in HIV-positive clients and how to promote better health habits.

Developing a Community HIV/AIDS Working Group to Coordinate and Solicit Care

Caring for HIV-infected patients and those overtly ill with AIDS is a long-term, difficult, time-consuming task, which will involve many people in the community besides the CMHC staff and a physician or two. The optimism for quick discovery of an effective vaccine or curative treatment has largely disappeared.

Each local community needs to create a community working group to coordinate care and to support those who work with HIV-infected persons. The CMHC is a logical organization to sponsor and host such a group. This group should include individuals from organizations that provide care or are affected by AIDS (usually a physician caring for AIDS patients), a representative from the local medical society, a local hospital administrator, a pharmacist handling AIDS drugs, and social service workers and volunteers from organizations providing services to AIDS patients.

This group can meet, perhaps monthly, to share ideas and problems about caring for AIDS patients in the community and to seek assistance from the political establishment when it is appropriate. The group can serve as a source of information about AIDS for the community and provide a forum for the expression of concern and the resolution of fear among citizens. The CMHC, with assistance from primary care physicians, can be the focus of the effort by the community to deal with the HIV epidemic.

Developing a Community HIV Working Group

- Recognize the complexity of caring for AIDS patients.
- Involve many individuals and community organizations.
- Host an AIDS "working group" or attend an existing one.
- Include a physician, pharmacist, hospital administrator, and representatives of all organizations and agencies providing assistance to AIDS patients.
- Meet to share ideas and provide mutual support.
- Provide a forum for community concerns.
- Provide a resource for AIDS educational efforts.

In summary, the list shows some of the steps that a CMHC can take to involve the community in responding to HIV disease. If such a group already exists in the community, then the CMHC can become an active participant. A community HIV working group enables agency staff to stay publicly associated with local physicians and other providers of care to assist clients in gaining access to the best available care.

Review Questions

1. How can CMHC staff best facilitate a client's HIV/AIDS medical treatment?

2. What are two ways to appeal to a physician to provide care to an HIV-infected client?

3. What are some of the most important reasons to participate in a community HIV working group?

References and Suggested Readings

Bresolin, L.B., Rinaldi, R.C., Henning, J.J., Harvey, L.K., Hendee, W.R., & Schwarz, M.R. (1990). Attitudes of U.S. primary care physicians about HIV disease and AIDS. *AIDS Care, 2*(2), 117–125.

Curtis, J.R., Paauw, D.S., Wenrich, M.D., Caroline, J.D., & Ramsey, P.G. (1995). Physicians' ability to provide initial primary care to the HIV-infected patient. *Archives of Internal Medicine, 155*(15), 1613–1618.

Gerbert, B., Maguire, B.T., Bleecker, T., Coates, T.J., & McPhee, S.J. (1991). Primary care physicians and AIDS: Attitudinal and structural barriers to care. *Journal of the American Medical Association, 266*(20), 2837–2842.

Gleeson, C.J., Havron, A., & Wadland, W.C. (1994). Family physician management of HIV and AIDS: A Vermont study. *Journal of Family Practice, 39*(1), 50–54.

Green, J., & Arno, P.S. (1990). The "Medicaidization" of AIDS: Trends in the financing of HIV-related medical care. *Journal of the American Medical Association, 264*(10), 1261–1266.

Sadovsky R. (1989). HIV-infected patients: A primary care challenge. *American Family Practice, 40*(3), 121–128.

Samuels, M.E., Shi, L., Stoskoph, C.H., Richter, D.L., Baker, S.L., & Sy, F.S. (1993). Incentives for physicians to treat HIV-seropositive patients: Results of a statewide survey. *Southern Medical Journal, 86*(4), 403–408.

Van Dyke, R.B. (1991). Pediatric human immunodeficiency virus infection and the acquired immunodeficiency syndrome: A health care crisis of children and families. *American Journal of Diseases of Children, 145*(5), 529–532.

Wartenberg, A.A. (1991). HIV disease in the intravenous drug user: Role of the primary care physician. *Journal of General Internal Medicine, 6* (suppl1), S35–S40.

Wofsey, C.B. (1988). AIDS care: Providing care for the HIV infected. *Journal of Acquired Immune Deficiency Syndromes, 1*(3), 274–283.

Part III

Mental Health
Interventions for HIV

Chapter 9

Neuropsychological Functioning in HIV Disease

Timothy L. Boaz, Ph.D.

Overview

This chapter reviews information on changes in neuropsychological functioning in persons with HIV disease. Information is presented about the prevalence, course, and symptoms of neuropsychological disorders associated with HIV disease.

Knowledge of symptoms of neuropsychological disorders that occur in persons with HIV disease will help community mental health center (CMHC) staff to understand the behavior of their clients who may be experiencing symptoms of such disorders and to make appropriate referrals for evaluation and treatment. The information will also be useful for staff who are assisting clients to make decisions about housing, employment, finances, and other personal arrangements.

Learning Objectives

1. To identify the three major types of disorders that cause neuropsychological impairment in HIV disease.

2. To recognize major differences between dementia and delirium in persons with HIV disease.

3. To identify the three major symptoms of dementia associated with HIV disease.

4. To recognize when to make referrals for neuropsychological assessment.

Outline

   I. Causes of Neuropsychological Disorders in HIV Disease
      A. Focal brain impairment
      B. Indirect diffuse CNS compromise
      C. Direct CNS infection by HIV

  II. Frequency of Neuropsychological Disorders in HIV Disease

 III. Delirium and Dementia in HIV Disease
      A. Diagnosis and features of delirium
      B. Intervention with delirium
      C. Diagnosis and features of dementia

 IV. Course of Neuropsychological Impairment in HIV Disease
      A. Early symptoms of HIV-related dementia
         1. Cognitive
         2. Behavioral
         3. Motor
      B. Neurological signs in late-stage HIV-related dementia

  V. Diagnostic Issues in HIV-Related Dementia
      A. "Functional" versus "organic" disorders
      B. Depression versus dementia
      C. Assessment techniques
      D. Referral for assessment

 VI. Management Issues in HIV-Related Dementia
      A. Pharmacological management
      B. Behavioral management

VII. Conclusion

Causes of Neuropsychological Disorders in HIV Disease

A surprising finding in the early years of the HIV epidemic was that some persons diagnosed with AIDS complained of difficulty with cognition. Later, it was recognized that a substantial number of persons with HIV infection develop a significant and, in some cases, profound and progressive loss of cognitive ability (Price, et. al., 1988).

HIV-related cognitive impairment can be caused by three different types of neurological problems.

Causes of Neuropsychological Disorders in HIV Disease

- Focal Brain Impairment
    - Cancer
        - Lymphoma
        - Other tumors
    - Toxoplasmosis
    - Cerebrovascular accidents (strokes)

- Indirect Diffuse Central Nervous System (CNS) Compromise
        - Opportunistic viral and fungal infections of brain
            - Progressive multifocal leukoencephalopathy
        - Metabolic abnormality
            - Thyroid
            - Electrolyte imbalance
        - Drug toxicity or withdrawal

- Direct CNS Infection by HIV

Some persons with AIDS develop cancer of the brain, most frequently lymphoma, or experience strokes. These types of disorders are "focal" in that they affect specific, limited areas of the brain. The effects of the focal lesion on a person's cognitive abilities are dependent on the type, location, and size of the brain area affected. The symptoms can be varied. These focal lesions occur in a minority of cases of HIV disease with cognitive impairment.

Originally, it was thought that the neuropsychological deficits found in association with AIDS were caused by the opportunistic infections and illnesses that were a result of a compromised immune system. Several of these conditions have direct effects on the brain. For example, toxoplasmosis is a focal infection that can occur in the brain. Others, such as drug side effects or metabolic abnormalities, may have more indirect effects on brain functioning. These types of neurological disorders are referred to as "indirect" causes of brain dysfunction in HIV disease because, in these cases, the brain impairment is not directly caused by HIV.

The majority of cases of neuropsychological impairment in persons with HIV infection are caused by the direct infection of the brain by HIV. It is not known exactly how the virus impairs brain functioning, but it appears that the virus does not directly infect the neurons. Rather, it appears that the virus infects other cells that play a supporting role in brain functioning. These infected cells may release substances that damage or impair the functioning of the neurons causing cognitive impairment.

Frequency of Neuropsychological Disorders in HIV Disease

Although there has been some debate as to how frequently neuropsychological disorders are found in persons with asymptomatic HIV disease, for those persons diagnosed with AIDS, approximately two-thirds will experience significant cognitive impairment before death, and 30 percent will show other symptoms of neurological disease. Autopsy studies have shown that brain abnormalities are found in 70–90 percent of persons who have died from AIDS. These data indicate that it is probable that persons with HIV disease will experience some impairment of their cognitive functioning in the course of the disease. However, it is not clear how early one can expect to begin to experience problems with cognitive abilities.

Studies of the cerebrospinal fluid in persons with HIV disease have shown that the brain can be infected with HIV early in the course of the disease (Price et al., 1988). Some reports have indicated that as many as 10 percent of cases initially present with cognitive impairment as the first or only symptom of HIV infection. In 1987, Grant and colleagues (Grant et al., 1987) reported that, in a small sample of asymptomatic HIV-positive clients, 44 percent performed abnormally on a battery of neuropsychological tests. These results caused concern about whether to protect the public, there should be mandatory HIV testing of persons in sensitive, high-stress, or high safety-risk jobs. However, numerous recent studies have shown that, among persons who are HIV-positive but otherwise asymptomatic, only a few appear to experience cognitive impairment that has a significant effect on their ability to work (van Gorp et al., 1993).

Delirium and Dementia in HIV Disease

As already mentioned, in cases where a person develops a brain tumor or other focal neurological condition that affects only a specific part of the brain, the person may develop specific, limited types of problems with cognition. More commonly, however, widespread areas of the brain will be affected and the effects on cognition will be more general. In these cases, there are two distinct sets of symptoms (or syndromes) that may be seen. These are referred to as "delirium" and "dementia."

Delirium in HIV Disease

- Disturbance of consciousness
- Reduced ability to focus, sustain, or shift attention
- Change in cognition (not as a result of dementia)
    - Memory impairment
    - Disorientation
    - Language disturbance
    - Perceptual disturbance

- Features:
    - Rapid onset
    - Fluctuating course
    - Brief duration

Although delirium occurs less frequently than does dementia in HIV disease, it is important to recognize because it may indicate the presence of a serious medical problem that requires immediate treatment. Delirium is sometimes also called an "acute confusional state." The usual symptoms of delirium, taken from the diagnostic criteria of the *Diagnostic and Statistical Manual of Mental Disorders,* 4th ed. (DSM-IV) (American Psychiatric Association, 1994) are outlined above. In delirium, the person's level of consciousness is affected (sometimes referred to as "clouding"). Symptoms that indicate clouding of consciousness include disorganized thinking and a reduced ability to maintain or appropriately shift attention. Disorganized thinking may be indicated by rambling, irrelevant, or incoherent speech.

If the person has a reduced ability to maintain attention, he or she may appear very easily distracted, and questions may have to be repeated frequently.

Difficulties with shifting attention may be indicated if the person does not respond appropriately when spoken to or if he or she keeps giving the same answer to questions whether or not it is appropriate (perseverates). Other symptoms of delirium include drowsiness, hallucinations or delusions, disruption of the sleep-wake cycle, agitation, disorientation as to time or place, and memory impairment.

Delirium usually develops rapidly and may last for only a few hours or days. The severity of symptoms may fluctuate significantly over the course of the day. Persons with delirium often show evidence of emotional disturbance. The symptoms of delirium are often experienced as frightening.

Interventions with Delirium in HIV Disease

■ Obtain a complete medical evaluation.

–Treat all treatable conditions.

■ Use psychoactive medication cautiously.

–Minimize CNS depressant medications.

–Beware that high-potency neuroleptics may cause neuroleptic malignant syndrome.

■ Provide psychosocial interventions.

–Explain the condition to the patient.

–Provide a quiet, low-distraction environment.

–Enable frequent contact with small number of well-known persons.

–Provide frequent orienting cues.

–Restore the usual sleep cycle.

Interventions for persons exhibiting symptoms of delirium are listed above. Persons who show signs of delirium should be referred for medical evaluation so that the immediate cause of the delirium can be identified and treated. In most cases, the delirium will resolve with proper treatment of the medical problem. In addition to proper medical treatment, the management of delirium may include psychosocial interventions, such as providing a quiet environment for the client which is relatively free of distracting stimuli. Frequent contact with one or two well-known persons and providing support and frequent orienting cues may help to reduce fears and improve orientation. A normal sleep-wake cycle should be restored, and sedation may be used to reduce agitation.

Dementia in HIV Disease

- Demonstrable impairment of short- and long-term memory
- One of the following:
    - Aphasia (language disturbance)
    - Apraxia (impaired ability to carry out motor activities)
    - Agnosia (impaired recognition of objects)
    - Impaired executive functioning (impaired abstraction, judgment, planning, etc.)
- Interference with normal, daily activities
- Signs and symptoms occurring not only during delirium
- Features:
    - Slow onset
    - Progressive, chronic course
    - Longer duration

Dementia is more common than delirium in persons with HIV disease. The *DSM-IV* diagnostic criteria for dementia are listed above. The most important symptom of dementia is an impairment of short-term and long-term memory. A person with dementia also will show a change in at least one other area of cognitive ability. These include the ability to engage in abstract thinking, to exercise appropriate judgment, to use language, to carry out skilled movements, or to recognize familiar objects. The symptoms must represent a significant decline from the person's previous level of cognitive functioning, and the symptoms must be severe enough that they interfere with the ability to carry out normal daily activities. In contrast to delirium, dementia usually develops slowly over months or years, and the symptoms do not fluctuate as significantly and rapidly as they do in delirium.

HIV disease is certainly not the only medical problem that can cause dementia or delirium; there are many others. However, most of these other causes of dementia and delirium occur more frequently in elderly persons. Whenever a relatively young person shows a clear decline in cognitive ability in the absence of a known medical cause, HIV infection should be considered as a possibility. On the other hand, it should not be assumed that dementia or delirium occurring in elderly persons is not attributable to HIV infection. Because HIV does sometimes infect elderly persons, it should be considered in the evaluation of dementia and delirium in the elderly.

Course of Neuropsychological Impairment in HIV Disease

Symptoms of HIV-related cognitive impairment vary with the stage of the disease. The course of neuropsychological disorders is shown here.

Course of Neuropsychological Disorders in HIV Disease

- A few cases have acute onset with delirium, psychosis, or mania.
- Most cases of HIV-related dementia have slow, progressive onset.
- Progression of symptoms is slow at first, rapid later.
- "Higher" brain functions are not affected until late in the illness.

In some cases, patients may experience symptoms of delirium at the time of seroconversion (when the blood begins to show evidence of HIV infection) resulting from an acute infection of the brain. However, since the immune system is not yet impaired, the body is usually able to recover from this infection and the delirium spontaneously subsides.

In most cases of HIV disease, as long as the person is otherwise asymptomatic, he or she is not likely to exhibit symptoms of cognitive impairment. However, a few patients will experience some cognitive decline before the onset of other AIDS symptoms. As AIDS symptoms begin to appear, the likelihood of cognitive impairment increases. At first, this impairment will be mild and hardly noticeable. Over time the symptoms may become more severe. The rate of decline in cognitive ability in persons with HIV-related dementia varies considerably from case to case. It appears that the rate of deterioration is slow at first but more rapid in the later stages of the disease. There are no known ways of predicting how fast the symptoms may progress for an individual case. In some cases, persons with AIDS never show any significant cognitive decline.

Early Symptoms of HIV-Related Dementia

- Cognitive:
    - Forgetfulness
    - Loss of concentration
    - Confusion
    - Slowness of thought

- Behavioral:
    - –Apathy
    - –Withdrawal
    - –Dysphoric mood

- Motor:
    - –Loss of balance
    - –Leg weakness
    - –Impaired handwriting

The most common symptoms of early HIV-related dementia can be organized into three categories: cognitive, behavioral, and motor. All of these symptoms do not necessarily appear in all cases of HIV-related dementia, and persons are likely to have more difficulty with some of these problems than with others.

Cognitive symptoms of early HIV-related dementia mainly involve difficulty with memory and concentration along with mental slowing. The affected persons may forget appointments or may need to keep lists to remember things. They may lose track of conversations, or they may need additional time and effort to organize their thoughts or to complete daily tasks.

Behavioral symptoms include apathy and depressed mood. Clients may appear less interested in work or social activities. They may become withdrawn, tire more easily, and may appear depressed or irritable.

Motor symptoms include problems with balance and coordination. Patients may trip more frequently while walking or may drop things more often. They may complain of leg weakness, or their handwriting may become sloppy.

Neurological Signs in Late-Stage HIV-Related Dementia

- Psychomotor retardation
- Mutism (inability to speak)
- Severe dementia
- Ataxia (difficulty walking)
- Hypertonia (rigidity)
- Incontinence
- Tremor

In the later stages of HIV-related dementia, the patient can experience more severe symptoms, including disruption of higher cognitive functioning such as the use of language. The patient's speech may become slow, and there may be difficulty finding words. Problem solving and judgment may be quite impaired.

Diagnostic Issues in HIV-Related Dementia

Issues in Diagnosis and Management of Neuropsychological Disorders in HIV Disease

■ Frequency

  –Dementia is a presenting symptom in 5–15 percent of cases of AIDS.

  –60–70% of patients show moderate dementia before death.

  –30% of patients have focal neurological disease in the late stages of AIDS.

■ Diagnosis

  –Organic mental disorders often appear like "functional" psychiatric disorders.

  –Early cognitive impairment may be subtle and may be present before appearance of neurologic signs.

  –Cognitive impairment may be present even if all neurodiagnostic tests are normal.

■ Dementia versus Depression

  –Symptoms of depression and subcortical dementia are similar.

  –Co-morbidity of depression and HIV disease is high.

  –Indications of depression are:

    –Depressive cognitions (worthlessness and guilt);

    –History of previous psychiatric dysfunction;

    –Poor or variable test-taking motivation;

    –Improvement with antidepressant medication.

Mental healthcare workers should keep several issues in mind when working with persons with HIV disease. First, organic mental disorders often mimic "functional" psychiatric disorders. Among the frequent symptoms of HIV-related dementia are depressed or irritable mood. Hallucinations or delusions may be seen in episodes of delirium. Thus, persons with HIV disease may appear to be depressed, manic, or schizophrenic. Since there are a number of ways that HIV can disrupt the functioning of the brain, various combinations of symptoms are possible. The appearance of functional psychiatric symptoms in persons with HIV disease should be assumed to be a result of organic factors unless demonstrated to be otherwise.

The changes in mental status that occur in the early stages of HIV disease are often subtle and may be present for some time before clear-cut neurological signs become apparent. These early changes are often difficult to detect. If one suspects that a person with HIV disease has some cognitive impairment or indications of dementia or delirium, that person should be referred to a psychologist or psychiatrist for further evaluation.

Determining whether a person is experiencing dementia or depression or both is a difficult diagnostic problem. There are two reasons for this difficulty. First, HIV-positive persons are likely to exhibit clinical depression. Second, two of the symptoms of HIV-related dementia are apathy and depressed mood.

Because the two disorders have different treatment and management implications, an accurate diagnosis is important. Community mental health workers serve an important role in observing the behavior of clients and in making clinical observations. Their knowledge of the client's history can be valuable to the psychiatrist, physician, or psychologist making the diagnosis.

There are a number of important factors to be considered in making this distinction. Persons with depression and persons with dementia are both likely to appear depressed, apathetic, helpless, and withdrawn. However, persons with depression are more likely to express feelings of guilt, worthlessness, and hopelessness, as well as suicidal ideation, than are persons with dementia. Persons with depression are more likely to have a history of depression before the diagnosis of HIV disease. They are more likely to show improvement when treated with antidepressant medication, whereas persons with HIV-related dementia may show improvement in their depressionlike symptoms in response to treatment with psychostimulants such as Ritalin or dextroamphetamine. On mental status testing, persons with depression are more likely to have poor or variable test-taking motivation (for example, they respond "I don't know" frequently). Persons with dementia are more likely to attempt a response but simply be incorrect.

There are three major types of assessment procedures used to examine persons with possible HIV-related neuropsychological disorders. These will be briefly described along with some of the advantages and disadvantages of each.

Assessment Techniques in HIV Disease

■ Neurological tests and procedures

--Highly specific

--Not necessarily sensitive to dementia

--Useful for ruling out certain neurological conditions

■ Neuropsychological testing

--Very sensitive

--Time-consuming and expensive

■ Mental status examination

--Brief and rapid

--Provides global assessment

--Lacking in sensitivity

--Lacking in comprehensiveness

Great advances have been made in neurological tests and procedures in recent years, particularly in the area of neuroimaging techniques. Electroencephalograms (EEGs) and computed tomography (CT) magnetic resonance imaging (MRI), and positron emission tomography (PET) scans all produce valuable information about the physical status of the human brain. However, these methods are not helpful in detecting the presence of direct infection of the brain by HIV or in determining when dementia is present. Since most cases of HIV-related dementia are the result of the direct infection of the brain by the virus, it is possible for the neurological examination and all neuroimaging tests such as CT or MRI scans to be normal, even if clinically significant cognitive impairment is present. On the other hand, these neuroimaging methods are very useful in detecting the presence of other possible brain illnesses or injuries, such as tumors, abscesses, or strokes that can and do occur in persons with HIV disease.

The most frequently used method for detecting the presence of clinically significant dementia is the brief mental status examination, such as the Mini-Mental State Exam (MMSE) (Folstein, Folstein, and McHugh, 1975). This test can be given quickly and requires little formal training to administer. It is most useful in identifying cases with moderately severe, global cognitive impairment. However, because it is brief, the MMSE has the drawback of lacking sensitivity; that is, the items may not be difficult enough to detect dementia, particularly in highly intelligent persons. The MMSE, and other similar tests, also lacks comprehensiveness because the person may be experiencing decline in an area of cognitive ability that is not measured well by the test. Thus, this test may not be useful for screening for cognitive impairment in persons with possible HIV-related dementia, particularly if the patient had relatively high premorbid cognitive ability and is experiencing relatively mild HIV-related cognitive impairment. If the MMSE suggests cognitive impairment, the patient should be referred for neuropsychological evaluation. If the MMSE fails to detect impairment, but the patient or family describe behavior suggesting significant cognitive impairment, the patient should be referred for neuropsychological evaluation.

Neuropsychological testing is conducted by clinical psychologists who are trained in assessment techniques for detecting the presence of cognitive impairment. Neuropsychological testing usually involves the measurement of various specific cognitive abilities. The client's performance on such tests is compared with the usual performance obtained from persons of comparable age and educational backgrounds. These tests are generally sensitive to the type of impairment seen in HIV-related dementia; however, most of the tests must be administered individually by a doctoral-level psychologist trained in neuropsychological assessment, and the tests are time-consuming and, therefore, expensive. Thus, neuropsychological testing is not feasible for routine assessments in most cases. However, referral for neuropsychological assessment should be made in cases where cognitive impairment may exist.

Clinicians should be vigilant for indicators of the presence of cognitive impairment. Such indicators may include signs of forgetfulness, such as double-booking or forgetting appointments; changes in personality, such as apathy, withdrawal, or increased irritability; and slowed response time and difficulty with complex problem solving, such as difficulty with driving. Observations of impaired cognition by friends or relatives can be extremely helpful. Complaints of impaired cognition by the patient are often strongly associated with depressed mood, and such complaints should be taken seriously and investigated for depression and dementia.

Management Issues in HIV-Related Dementia

Pharmacological Management

Pharmacological management of HIV-related dementia can involve two approaches. Treatment may be aimed at the cause of the cognitive impairment itself or it may be designed to ameliorate symptoms of the disorder.

As described above, cognitive impairment in HIV may be resulting directly from HIV infection or it may be the result of other indirect factors. In the case of cognitive impairment directly caused by HIV infection, it has been shown (e.g., Schmitt et al., 1988) that, in some cases, symptoms of HIV-related dementia abate with antiviral therapy. Thus, treatment of the dementia occurs along with treatment of the HIV infection itself. When the cognitive impairment is a result of other, indirect factors, cognitive impairment may abate with successful treatment of the underlying cause of the cognitive impairment.

Other symptoms that can co-occur with HIV-related dementia may be treated symptomatically. For example, associated symptoms of depression may be treated with antidepressant medications such as the selective serotonin reuptake inhibitors (SSRIs); agitation may be treated with haloperidol; mania may be treated with lithium or valproic acid; lethargy may be treated with amphetamine or methylphenidate; and lastly, trazodone, doxepin, or amitriptyline may be used for sedation (and some antidepressant effect).

It has been reported that persons with HIV-related cognitive impairment may be more sensitive to both therapeutic effects and side effects of psychotropic medications (Zeifert, Leary, and Boccellari, 1996). Thus, it is recommended that such patients be started at lower than usual dosages of these medications, and that changes to medication regimens be gradual.

Refer to Bartlett (1996) and Fernandez and Levy (1994) for more thorough and authoritative discussions of the psychopharmacology of HIV-related dementia.

Behavioral Management

Several authors have outlined suggestions for behavioral management of difficulties associated with HIV-related dementia. One excellent source is Buckingham and van Gorp (1988) from which many of the following suggestions are drawn. These strategies consist of both compensatory behaviors and environmental engineering.

To compensate for forgetfulness, persons with HIV-related cognitive impairment can be encouraged to use appointment books or calendars to keep track of scheduled events and to use a logbook or journal to remind them of events that have already occurred. They can use notebooks to keep lists of to-be-remembered items. Leaving reminder notes in strategic places may serve as an effective memory aid.

For problems with attention and concentration, patients may be encouraged to limit distractions (such as radio or television) when they need to attend to something. Working on one thing at a time, breaking large tasks into smaller, more manageable tasks, and allowing more time for completion of tasks can aid in attention and concentration.

To cope with slowness of thinking, patients should be encouraged to schedule more time for completion of tasks and should avoid tasks for which speed of performance is essential.

It is helpful to maintain a consistent, predictable environment and schedule. Keeping stressors to a minimum is also helpful.

In the case of progressive dementia, as the symptoms become more severe, the focus will shift from assisting the person with cognitive impairment in using compensatory strategies to a strategy of providing more support in the person's environment. Intervention may also focus more on the person's caregiver. It is important for such caregivers to have an adequate understanding of the nature of symptoms they are observing. For example, the moderately to severely impaired patient may be distractible and impulsive and may manifest inappropriate behavior or angry outbursts. It is important for the caregiver to recognize these as symptoms of the disorder, rather than seeing them as volitional behavior on the part of the patient and taking them personally. In such cases, redirecting the patient's behavior or distracting the patient may be a more effective intervention than confrontation.

Conclusion

Most persons with HIV disease will experience cognitive impairment during the course of the disease. Symptoms of neuropsychological disorders in HIV disease are often mistakenly interpreted as symptoms of other psychiatric disorders. Because the presence of neuropsychological disorders in HIV disease has important implications for treatment and management, community mental health workers play an important role in identifying cases in which cognitive impairment is present and in referring such cases for appropriate evaluation.

Review Questions

1. Identify three observations that would help you recognize delirium in someone with HIV disease.

2. Describe a major feature that distinguishes between dementia and delirium.

3. Name the three major types of neurological disease that cause neuropsychological impairment in HIV disease.

References and Suggested Readings

American Psychiatric Association. (1994). *Diagnostic and Statistical Manual of Mental Disorders* (4th ed.). Washington, D.C.

Bartlett, J.G. (1996). *Pocket Book of Infectious Disease Therapy.* Baltimore: Williams & Wilkins.

Boccelari, A., & Zeifert, P. (1993). Management of neurobehavioral impairment in HIV-1 infection. *Psychiatric Clinics of North America, 17,* 183–203.

Buckingham, S.L., & van Gorp, W.G. (1988). AIDS-dementia complex: Implications for practice. *Journal of Contemporary Social Work, 69,* 371–375.

Buckingham, S.L., & Van Gorp, W.G. (1994). HIV-associated dementia: A clinician's guide to early detection, diagnosis, and intervention. *Families in Society: The Journal of Contemporary Human Services, 75,* 333–345.

Fernandez, F., & Levy, J.K. (1994). Psychopharmacology in HIV spectrum disorders. *Psychiatric Clinics of North America, 17,* 135–148.

Folstein, M.F., Folstein, S.E., & McHugh, P.R. (1975). Mini-Mental State: A practical method for grading the cognitive state of patients for the clinician. *Journal of Psychiatric Research, 12,* 189–198.

Glass, J.D., & Johnson, R.T. (1996). Human immunodeficiency virus and the brain. *Annual Review of Neuroscience, 19,* 1–26.

Grant, I., Atkinson, J.H., Hesselink, J.R., Kennedy, C.J., Richman, D.D., Spector, S.A., & McCutchan, J.A. (1987). Evidence for early central nervous system involvement in the acquired immunodeficiency syndrome (AIDS) and other human immunodeficiency virus (HIV) infections. *Annals of Internal Medicine, 107,* 828–836.

Greenwood, D.U. (1991). Neuropsychological aspects of AIDS dementia complex: What clinicians need to know. *Professional Psychology: Research and Practice, 22,* 407–409.

Maj, M. (1990). Psychiatric aspects of HIV-1 infection and AIDS. *Psychological Medicine, 20,* 547–563.

Mapou, R.L., & Law, W.A. (1994). Neurobehavioral aspects of HIV disease and AIDS: An update. *Professional Psychology: Research and Practice, 25,* 132–140.

Nadler, J.P., Greene, J., Himmelright, I., & Toney, J.F. (1995). Clinically significant human immunodeficiency virus infection in the elderly. *Infectious Diseases in Clinical Practice, 4*(4), 304–306.

Ochitill, H.N., & Dilley, J.W. (1988). Neuropsychiatric aspects of acquired immunodeficiency syndrome. In M.L. Rosenblum, R.M. Levy, & D.E. Dredesen (Eds.), *AIDS and the Nervous System.* 315–325. New York: Raven Press.

Perry, S.W. (1990). Organic mental disorders caused by HIV: Update on early diagnosis and treatment. *American Journal of Psychiatry, 147,* 696–710.

Price, R.W., Sidtis, J.J., Navia, B.A., Pumarola-Sune, T., & Ornitz, D.B. (1988). The AIDS dementia complex. In M.L. Rosenblum, R.M. Levy, & D.E. Dredesen (Eds.), *AIDS and the Nervous System.* (203–219). New York: Raven Press.

Price, R.W., Sidtis, J., & Rosenblum, M. (1988). The AIDS dementia complex: Some current questions. *Annals of Neurology, 23*(suppl), S27–S33.

Schmitt, F.A., Bigley, J.W., McKinnis, R., Logue, P.E., Evans, R.W., & Drucker, J.L. (1988). Neuropsychological outcome of zidovudine (AZT) treatment of patients with AIDS and AIDS-related complex. *New England Journal of Medicine, 319,* 1573–1578.

Sidtis, J.J., & Price, R.W. (1990). Early HIV-1 infection and the AIDS dementia complex. *Neurology, 40,* 323–326.

Stall, R., & Catania, J. (1994). AIDS risk behaviors among late middle-aged and elderly Americans. The National AIDS Behavioral Surveys. *Archives of Internal Medicine, 154*(1), 57–63.

Tross, S., & Hirsch, D.A. (1988). Psychological distress and neuropsychological complications of HIV. *American Psychologist, 43,* 929–934.

van Gorp, W.G., Hinkin, C., Satz, P., Miller, E., & D'Elia, L.F. (1993). Neuropsychological findings in HIV infection, encephalopathy, and dementia. In R.W. Parks, R.F. Zec, & R.S. Wilson (Eds.), *Neuropsychology of Alzheimer's Disease and Other Dementias.* New York: Oxford University Press.

Zeifert, P., Leary, M., & Boccellari, A. (1996). Treatment of cognitive impairment. *Focus: A Guide to AIDS Research and Counseling, 11*(3), 1–8.

Chapter 10

▪ Notifying Others of Seropositivity

Charles F. Clark, M.D., M.P.H.

Overview

This chapter prepares Community Mental Health Center (CMHC) staff to discuss HIV status with clients and to prepare clients to make decisions about telling other people. The importance of helping clients create emotional safety is stressed. This includes being able to discriminate between people who can help and be trusted and those who cannot; becoming comfortable about telling others; handling prejudice against persons with HIV disease; and locating support groups.

Learning Objectives

1. To distinguish between being HIV-seropositive and having AIDS.

2. To distinguish between "safe" and "unsafe" people to whom clients may disclose HIV status.

3. To identify possible negative reactions from others that a client may have to deal with when disclosing his or her HIV status.

4. To identify three ways in which a client may safeguard personal safety when choosing whether to disclose her or his HIV status.

Outline

I. The Meaning of Being HIV-Seropositive
   A. Infected with HIV
   B. May or may not be ill
   C. May or may not have AIDS
   D. Potentially infectious

II. Who Has the Right to Reveal a Person's HIV Status?

III. Helping Clients Make Decisions about Disclosing Their Status
   A. Telling people who need to know
   B. Educating the people that one chooses to tell
   C. Accepting sympathy and offers of help

IV. How to Tell Another Person That One Is HIV-Positive
   A. Choose an unhurried time
   B. Choose a private place
   C. Tell people one at a time
   D. Take a friend or counselor to help

V. Handling Discrimination against People Who Are HIV-Positive

VI. Locating Local HIV Support Groups

The Meaning of Being HIV-Seropositive

Not everyone exposed to a virus such as HIV becomes infected. A large number of virus particles must be introduced by a proper route for infection to take place. The hallmark of successful infection is the development of antibodies. A person who is HIV-seropositive, that is, who has antibodies to HIV, is infected with HIV.

Having a positive HIV test, commonly but incorrectly called the "AIDS test," means that the person has been infected with HIV. It does not mean that the person has AIDS. Typically, an HIV-infected person will not develop AIDS until at least five years have passed and frequently will not become seriously ill until ten to fourteen years have passed. A seropositive test result does not mean that the person is ill, cannot work, or is otherwise disabled.

What Does HIV-Seropositivity Mean?

- The person is infected with HIV.
- The person may or may not be ill.
- The person may or may not have AIDS.
- The person is potentially infectious to sexual partners, fetuses, partners who share injection drug paraphernalia, and anyone who accepts their blood, semen, or organ donations.

The list above summarizes the meaning of being HIV-positive. An HIV-positive person has been exposed to the virus and is infected with HIV; may or may not be ill or have AIDS; and is potentially infectious to sexual partners, fetuses, and injection drug-sharing partners.

Who Has the Right to Reveal a Person's HIV Status?

An individual's health condition is confidential information and, with rare exceptions, only the individual has the right to decide to reveal this information. For example, a staff person at a community mental health center does not have the right to divulge a client's HIV status without permission.

The Dilemma of Revealing HIV Status

- Health status is a person's own private information.
- Every person has a responsibility to protect the health of their fellow citizens.
- Ideally, this apparent conflict is resolved by the community helping the person and the person protecting the community.
- CMHC staff may help clients and the community to resolve this dilemma in ways that protect everyone.

HIV is an infectious disease; if the infection endangers the health of others, those persons have a legitimate claim to the information. In our society, our freedoms do not permit us to harm or threaten to harm others. This creates a dilemma in which the HIV-positive person's rights are weighed against the rights of people whose health may be endangered. As community mental health workers, we can help both clients and communities create an environment that protects everyone.

Helping HIV-Positive Clients Make Decisions about Disclosing Their Status

When a client is trying to decide whether to disclose her or his HIV status, it is important to remember that, in the United States, persons with HIV infection have sometimes been discriminated against in terrible ways. Seropositive persons are appropriately concerned about telling others of their infection and are likely to need help in making decisions about revealing their infection. They may not realize the importance of telling certain people and not telling others. A person with HIV infection, as with any person experiencing a life-threatening event, is under enormous, internally generated, emotional pressure to share the information with someone.

Telling People Who Need to Know

Community mental health center counselors may help clients sort out who must know and who is safe to trust with the information that they are HIV-positive. Each client's "need to know" list may differ from a "safe to tell" list. While the "need to know" category will vary with each person, it will generally include the following:

Need to Know

- Physician and other healthcare providers
- Mental health counselor
- Family and friends
- Religious advisor
- Employer (perhaps)
- Current sexual partners
- Former sexual partners
- Injection drug-sharing partners
- Plasmapheresis centers
- Blood banks
- Semen and organ banks

Generally, the people with whom that client is intimate or upon whom one relies for physical, emotional, and sometimes financial, support fall into the "need to know" category. This includes physicians, mental health counselors, family members, friends, religious advisors, and, perhaps, employers. It is essential that seropositive persons tell their physicians of the positive test. HIV infection damages several organ systems and, eventually, causes AIDS. It is simply not possible to provide good medical care if a physician does not know that a patient has HIV infection. Patients who cannot trust their physicians with the information should search for physicians they can trust. Even if not directly informed, nurses and technicians working with a physician will probably know a client's diagnosis because of the type of tests ordered and the medications used. It may be possible for a client to discuss how many people on the physician's staff must or will know of their status and receive reassurance of confidentiality.

Clients may decide to tell family members and close friends about their seropositive status. Some clients may fear rejection by family members. Counselors may need to reassure a client that most people, upon learning that a family member or friend has a serious illness, respond with concern and care. If they respond otherwise, it is generally because of fear. It may be possible to educate family and friends about HIV disease as part of the process of telling them about one's HIV status. Counselors may work with their clients on how best to set the stage for disclosure and to work through their fears about the reaction of their close associates. Many clients may want to tell their religious or spiritual advisors. It is the life work of these professionals to help persons and many religious denominations have conducted AIDS awareness training for their clergy. Many have developed special AIDS ministries. In some cases, a religious advisor may not sanction a particular type of behavior, but will express a sense of obligation to care for the individual. As with physicians, if one religious person seems patronizing or untrustworthy, another can usually be found.

Telling an employer of HIV seropositivity presents some difficulty. It is possible that the employer will terminate the seropositive employee or will discover some unrelated reason to dismiss the employee. This is a serious problem in our society which we have thus far failed to adequately address. Clients must assess their individual employers for themselves. It is impossible to give an assurance that employers will act appropriately, since the employers will consider the potential negative effects on their businesses. It may be possible to reassure an employer that employing someone who is HIV-positive is not dangerous to the public. Remember that discrimination based on HIV status is illegal. (See Chapter 3, "HIV and the Law.")

Although it is illegal and a violation of confidentiality, there is a chance that an employer will learn of the seropositivity through insurance reports, especially when the company is self-insured. Insurers have sometimes pressured employers to eliminate persons in high-risk categories by threatening to raise premiums or not renew a policy. Clients may wish to consult an attorney about their rights should this occur.

We all live in communities, patients and counselors alike, and we all have responsibilities to our communities. One of these responsibilities, a moral one, is to protect our fellow citizens from deadly infectious diseases. Likewise, the community has a responsibility to protect and care for those of its citizens who are ill, including those who are HIV-infected.

HIV infection is slow to cause disease but, eventually, is deadly. Those who are infected need assistance and, to get it, must take the risk of revealing the infection to others. Most people will respond with compassion and concern. Even those who may condemn the "group" of HIV/AIDS-infected persons will generally be compassionate to an individual who is ill.

Current and former sexual partners should be told of their exposure and possible infection and should be advised to be tested immediately. Telling them can be done directly, through a surrogate, or even anonymously. State laws vary on this subject. In the state of Florida, for example, it is illegal not to tell a current sexual partner that you are HIV-positive. Community mental health center counselors should check their state's law since many states now include HIV status under "duty to warn" laws. Contact tracing of past sexual partners has been a hotly debated topic in many states and, again, state laws vary.

All blood banks, plasmapheresis centers, semen banks, and organ banks must be notified if a donation was made within the last 10 years. All needle partners for the last 10 years must be notified and urged to obtain testing.

Educating the People One Chooses to Tell

Despite much information in the press and on television about HIV/AIDS, many people still do not understand the disease and its implications. Telling people that one is HIV-positive generally requires explaining what that means. Most people will be eager to learn about a disease that affects someone they know. It may be helpful to take pamphlets provided by public health agencies which give written information about the disease.

Accepting Sympathy and Offers of Help

Many people have difficulty accepting sympathy and offers of help. It is hard to view oneself as needing compassion and assistance from others. An HIV-positive person will find it easier to accept help if the helper is willing to listen to what the person needs. Assistance based on what a helping person "thinks" someone else needs is often perceived as interference or pushiness and is more likely to be rejected or resented. Counselors may be able to help clients learn to communicate their needs directly or to request that a helping person listen to what they have to say. Clients should tactfully refuse assistance that they do not perceive as useful.

How to Tell Others That One Is HIV-Positive

Telling others that one is HIV-positive is not significantly different from telling any other serious bad news. Most people feel the pain of the problem and immediately want to help and offer comfort. The following list shows some of the elements that can make telling bad news easier.

Telling Others That One Is HIV-Positive

- Choose an unhurried time.
- Choose a private place.
- Tell people one at a time.
- If a person is anxious about telling someone, he or she may take a friend or counselor to help out.

When and where to tell a person bad news is important. It is usually better to tell someone alone, in a quiet and unhurried setting. Give the person a chance to digest the news, consider the implications, and offer his or her support. People usually want to help, especially if they see themselves as a member of a special or confidential group that is helping a person with a socially difficult disease.

It is probably best that someone who is seropositive not tell a group of people all at once, unless the group was specifically organized by an experienced AIDS counselor. People in groups frequently respond differently than when approached individually. People in groups sometimes behave in unpredictable and even vicious ways, exhibiting behavior they may later regret and be unable to explain to themselves.

If a client is uncomfortable telling someone about his or her HIV status, CMHC staff may be able to help them find someone to go with them for support. The support person may offer reassurance against mistreatment or condemnation, although the chances of those reactions are remote. After being accompanied a time or two, the person may later be able to tell people alone.

When a person reveals their HIV status, people are often curious about how they contracted the disease. It is strictly up to the individual to decide to reveal any details about his or her behavior. Being frank and truthful may reduce the chance of inaccurate information spreading among family members and friends or in the general community. Many gay people, for example, find that when they take the risk of telling someone in the family that they are gay, the family member had guessed it years before but had not felt at liberty to bring it up. People like to be "in the know" and will appreciate the confidence implied by sharing information with them. Many people will be relieved to have information they already knew out in the open. Some people will pretend they knew and are, therefore, not surprised. Most people will be curious, not shocked, about how a person was exposed to the virus.

In some cases, people may think that a person with HIV contracted the disease from behavior that they, in fact, did not engage in. HIV-positive persons will have to decide how to handle false assumptions that they are drug users, are gay, or engage in unsafe sexual practices. Each person must develop a personal strategy for handling people's curiosity in a way that reinforces personal respect and safety. No one "owes" another person an explanation of their HIV status. Each person who is HIV-positive will decide with whom to share personal, confidential information. Clients may need to learn how to firmly but gently refuse to answer questions.

Upon disclosure of positive HIV status, the client may find that each person learning the news needs time to handle their own anxiety and grief about the possibility of losing a family member, friend, or employee to a terminal illness. It is natural for people to think of their own losses with a sense of dismay. The person who is HIV-positive can allow time for the person to adjust to the news and then can ask for the person's help with the difficult times that lie ahead. This reinforces the sense that you are facing this loss together and redirects the focus to fighting the disease. The following list shows some common reactions that people exhibit upon being told bad news.

Possible Reactions to Being Told

- Concern and compassion
- Readiness to help
- Appreciation to be confided in
- Willingness to become part of a protective, confidential group

Handling Discrimination against People Who Are HIV-Positive

Discrimination against HIV/AIDS patients is a real problem in our society. People with HIV disease, like other people who are victims of discrimination, have to constantly make choices about whether to disclose their status. Telling can sometimes trigger reactions ranging from unpleasant to physically dangerous. The choice of whether to be silent, tell the truth, or actually lie in any given situation is always the individual's personal decision. One way to help clients decide is to have them ask themselves whether they can live with the consequences of telling the truth, lying, or remaining silent. The consequences, and the individual's tolerance for them, will vary. While one person may be willing to handle telling an HIV-phobic employer that he or she is HIV-positive, another person may need the job so badly that they cannot take any chance of losing the job. There are not any "right" answers about how to avoid discrimination, because people's circumstances vary so widely.

The following are guidelines for facing discrimination:

Facing Discrimination

- Help clients think about their options.
- Help clients rehearse how to handle the consequences of revealing their positive status, lying, or being silent.
- Encourage revealing HIV status openly and honestly only if a person feels ready to handle the expected consequences.
- Help people who prefer to tell the truth not to blame themselves if they are in a situation in which they dissemble or lie to avoid negative or even dangerous consequences.

HIV-seropositive clients should not expose themselves unnecessarily to discrimination. They should tell only those whom they feel will be helpful. Specifically, they should not tell people who have treated them badly in the past or people with a reputation for being vicious toward others. They should avoid people who are likely to "blame the victim." The best predictor of the future behavior of a person is their past behavior. With rare exceptions, good, compassionate people stay that way.

Generally, HIV-seropositive clients should tell only people with whom they have a personal relationship. Most strangers will be helpful and sympathetic but, without a personal relationship, it is difficult to predict what they will ultimately do with information about HIV status. It is pointless to tell people who cannot offer any emotional support or assistance and, because of the widespread discrimination in this country, it is best not to tell those who do not need to know.

Locating Local HIV Support Groups

One of the most useful things that can be done for an HIV-seropositive person is to take him or her to an AIDS support group. Many people are initially reluctant to attend because it is an unfamiliar place with a room full of strangers, and one does not know what to say or do. Accompanying the person to the first meeting makes him or her much more likely to attend. Over time, the support and information from the group will be invaluable for every person that attends. There is comfort in belonging, even if no one would choose to qualify for membership.

Attendance at HIV/AIDS Support Groups

- Encourage the client to attend.
- Personally take the client to the first meeting, if necessary.
- Support groups are sources of support and education.
- Start a support group if none exists in the area.
- Churches and community support organizations exist to assist those in need.
- Request community support (housing, coffee, funds) for the HIV/AIDS support group.
- The request for support will serve to educate about a problem in the community.

If there is not an HIV support group in the area, the CMHC staff can start one. Ask a church to provide the meeting place. Ask the Rotary Club to donate a coffee pot and pay for the weekly coffee. Churches and civic organizations exist to serve. Provide them an opportunity to do so. Ask for help expecting to get it and it will appear.

Review Questions

1. Does a person who is infected with HIV have AIDS?

2. What advice should be given to a client with HIV disease regarding how to identify someone who is safe to tell?

3. What are some of the positive reactions one might expect from people when they are told someone they care about is HIV-positive?

4. What should a client with HIV disease consider in making a decision to apply for work at a local hospital as an orderly?

5. Would a family gathering be the best setting for a client to tell a family member about his or her HIV status?

References and Suggested Readings

Centers for Disease Control and Prevention. (1995). Notification of syringe-sharing and sex part-ners of HIV-infected persons—Pennsylvania, 1993–1994. *Morbidity and Mortality Weekly Report, 44*(11), 202–204.

Geisecke, G.A., Ramstedt, K., Graneth, F., Ripa, T., Rado, G., & Westrell, M. (1991). Efficacy of partner notification for HIV infection. *Lancet, 338*(8775), 1096–1100.

Isaacman, S.H., & Closen, M.L. (1989). Notifying contacts of HIV-infected patients; Strategies to use until health agencies assume responsibility. *Postgraduate Medicine, 85*(7), 42–44, 53–55, 59.

Mansfield, S.J., & Singh, S. (1989). The general practitioner and human immunodeficiency virus infection: An insight into patients' attitudes. *Journal of the Royal College of General Practitioners, 39*(320), 104–105.

Perry, S., Fishman, B. , Jacobsberg, L., Young, J., & Francis, A. (1991). Effectiveness of psycho-educational interventions in reducing emotional distress after human immunodeficiency virus antibody testing. *Archives of General Psychiatry, 48*(2), 143–147.

Watters, J.K. (1995). HIV test results, partner notification, and personal conduct. *Lancet, 346*(8971), 326–327.

Chapter 11

Effects of Stress: The Relationship between Health and Stress

Martha A. Friedrich, Ph.D.

Overview

This chapter presents background information on the study of stress, the relationship between health and stress, and stress as it is experienced in the course of HIV disease. Stress management interventions including relaxation, cognitive restructuring, social support, and exercise are discussed.

Learning Objectives

1. To specify at least two ways in which stress affects immune functioning.
2. To identify high-stress points in HIV disease.
3. To describe at least three interventions for stress management.

Outline

I. Stress in Health and Illness
   A. Models and theories of stress

1. Fight or flight response
2. General adaptation syndrome
3. Stress and social contexts
4. Social Readjustment Rating Scale
5. Adaptive coping

B. Psychoneuroimmunology

II. Stress and HIV Infection

A. Stress at pre- and post-HIV antibody testing

B. Stress in asymptomatic HIV-positive individuals

C. Stress among persons with AIDS

III. Stress Management Interventions

A. Relaxation training techniques

B. Cognitive restructuring

C. Enhancing social support

D. Importance of physical exercise

IV. Conclusion

Stress in Health and Illness

Many authors have pointed out the stress associated with being HIV-infected. Community mental health treatment staff should play an important role in assisting persons living with HIV or AIDS to reduce stress.

The concept that environmental stress can affect health is a very old one, but nineteenth century scientists focused on physical causes of disease and minimized or ignored the role of agents that could not be seen or measured. Interest in stress and health has revived since World War II. Current research supports the notion that people whose lives are disrupted have an increased risk of subsequently becoming physically or mentally ill.

Models and Theories of Stress

Fight or Flight Response

After years of study there is still no satisfactory definition of stress. In the 1930s, Walter Cannon studied the bodily effects of major emotions, including fear and anger. He identified physiological patterns of response to emergencies which prepare an organism to protect itself. This "fight or flight" response describes a level of physiological arousal associated with stress.

General Adaptation Syndrome

Hans Selye conducted further research on stress and identified the "general adaptation syndrome," which is a physiological response to an environmental demand. This response goes beyond the "fight or flight" reaction and includes a wide array of anatomical and biochemical changes in the body. Selye's postulate of a single, nonspecific physiological response to stressors has been replaced with the understanding that there are a variety of responses depending on the nature of the stressor. Responses to stressors can be physical (metabolic, hormonal), emotional (fear, anger, sadness), or both.

Stress and Social Contexts

In the 1960s, Barbara and Bruce Dohrenwend studied the prevalence and distribution of mental disorders in society using Selye's model of stress. They described stress reactions in terms of external stressors, factors that alleviate the effects of the stressor, and the individual's response to the stressor, including attempts to cope. Recent research in stress has emphasized coping and adaptation responses by the individual.

The Social Readjustment Rating Scale

While change is an inevitable part of life, too much change in too little time may be harmful to our health. Thomas Holmes and Richard Rahe studied the case histories of 5000 people and identified a long list of life events that seemed to precede major illnesses. Some of these events were positive or socially desirable and some were negative or socially undesirable. These events were then assigned a numerical score based on the amount, intensity, and length of readjustment it took for each life event on the list. This scaling system, called the Social Readjustment Rating Scale, has been used to predict susceptibility to illness.

By adding up the adjustment values for each life event experienced, a person can obtain a life-change score. Those who have a high life-change score are much more likely to contract an illness. Studies using this rating scale have shown that scores over 300 points are associated with an 80 percent chance of having a serious physical or emotional illness during the next two years. Scores between 150 and 300 are associated with a 50:50 chance of subsequent serious illness, and with scores below 150 the chances are about one in three. Major illness and the death of family members are high sources of stress.

The stress of life changes can be managed by understanding and anticipating the necessary readjustment. Knowing that an event listed on the Social

Readjustment Rating Scale is going to occur should lead an individual to expect stress and engage in whatever stress management techniques work for him or her. It is important to remember that many of the events on the list are viewed as positive changes. Nevertheless, the required adjustment takes its toll.

Adaptive Coping

A different approach to the relationship between stress and illness has been proposed by Antomonsky. He argues that because stress is so common, the odd fact is the number of people who seldom become ill. This approach leads to a focus on the adaptive coping engaged in by most people.

Human beings are not passive witnesses of events and experiences. Events have different meanings for different people. Social factors, like genetic or viral ones, play a role in the inception and maintenance of disease. If the events are perceived as challenging (stressful), they generate adaptive coping devices. People vary in the skill they use to cope with challenges, just as the events themselves vary. All of this variability leads to the different courses of illness for different individuals.

Once disease and illness occur, they too become experiences with which the person must cope. Factors that determine individual responses to disease include whether the disease comes on abruptly or gradually, is treatable, carries with it a special stigma, or requires hospitalization. A combination of high life event scores plus an unsuccessful coping response is especially potent in depressing immunological defenses.

Psychoneuroimmunology

Since the 1980s, interest in the interrelationship between biological and psychological systems has led to a new field of study called psychoneuroimmunology. As emotions, particularly stress-related emotions such as fear and anger, produce biochemical changes in the brain, immune function has been shown to change. Researchers are also studying the effects of immune status on psychological well-being.

The role of stress has been investigated both as a risk factor for the onset of a disease (e.g., peptic ulcer, hypertension) and as a risk factor in maintaining or exacerbating diseases such as rheumatoid arthritis and asthma. HIV research has focused more on this latter relationship. Stressors have been shown to enhance an individual's vulnerability to infectious diseases and delay recovery from physical illness.

In addition to documenting incidence or maintenance of disease associated with stress, researchers have sought specific underlying mechanisms by looking directly at immunological functions. For example, bereavement has been shown to depress lymphocyte functions as well as to modify hormonal responses (Calabrese, Kling, and Gold, 1987). Lymphocytes are some of the principal cells of the immune system. Psychological feelings of helplessness are associated with a higher incidence of cancer, and it is suggested that a depressed immune system is the mediating factor. Combinations of neurotransmitters and psychotropic medications can suppress immune response.

Several psychological variables, including depression, perceived loss of control, and feelings of helplessness have been associated with altered immune functioning. Individuals have been shown to be more vulnerable to infectious illness after major life stressors as well as after chronic minor stressors (Cohen and Williamson, 1991; Kiecolt-Glaser and Glaser, 1988).

In addition to the direct effects of stress on the immune system through brain-mediated physiological processes, there may be some indirect effects through associated behavior changes. Medication, lack of sleep, smoking, and drug and alcohol use are known to have immunosuppressive effects. Regular aerobic exercise has been shown to improve immune functioning.

Physical illness may cause depressive symptoms not only as a psychological reaction to the illness, but also as an expression of the immune system's efforts to protect the body. Fatigue, like fever, can be regulated by the immune system in its efforts to fight disease. Various neurotransmitters and central nervous system (CNS)-controlled hormones (such as insulin and testosterone) have specific receptor sites through which they affect the functional activity of lymphocytes. These are direct links between the CNS and the immune system. The thymus, which is central to CD4 (T-cell) regulation, also produces hormones as part of the neuroendocrine system. Brain activity is affected by immunologic responses.

Stress and HIV Infection

The HIV spectrum spans the time from initial infection, through the testing and diagnosis process, to serious illness and death. Throughout this time, most people learn to manage the stress of having the infection, but there are certain crisis points at which the stress becomes more difficult to handle. Some significant life-change events can be expected among those with HIV disease. Because of the way that the disease is transmitted, many people with HIV infection, especially gay men and injecting drug users, also know others who are infected. Multiple bereavement, also called bereavement overload, occurs when an individual is grieving the deaths of more than one person close to him or her. Such individuals are likely to experience an increase in psychological stress or substance abuse.

Stress at Pre- and Post-HIV Antibody Testing

Making the decision to have an HIV antibody test may be very stressful. At this time the individual acknowledges that there is some risk of infection because of past behavior. If the person has been denying or minimizing the risk, the decision to take a test is a decision to discontinue that denial. It may take several days to receive the results of the test and the wait may be very stressful. Many people will have the test but not want to know the results. Perhaps, at that time, they decide that denial is more comfortable than the truth. While anxiety levels are higher for those awaiting test results than for the general population, those who find out that they are not HIV-infected report anxiety below the norm six months after the test. Those who receive positive results and those who choose not to know their results are still more anxious than the norm six months after the test (Huggins et al., 1991).

Stress in Asymptomatic HIV-Positive Individuals

Eventually, the level of distress for those who learn that they are HIV-positive subsides. Realizing that there can be a long time before symptoms begin, people adjust to life with the virus. Many report anxiety or panic, however, when colds or fever develop, and most will report increasing concern with health status. The coping responses reported by these individuals are similar to, and as effective as, those of their seronegative counterparts. However, HIV infection may make some individuals more reactive to high levels of stress than similarly stressed noninfected individuals.

Any new negative changes in health status will be stressful for the HIV-infected individual. These include falling CD4 counts, beginning antiretroviral therapy, and developing HIV-related symptoms. Psychosocial issues, including changing sex and drug behavior and notifying others of HIV status, may also be sources of stress.

In early studies, it was often observed that people beginning to develop the early signs of AIDS experienced more stress than those with full-blown AIDS (Tross and Hirsch, 1988). Those with only early signs reported that they were always "waiting for the other shoe to drop" and that the uncertainty was the source of their distress. Many people reported it was a relief to finally get an unequivocal diagnosis of AIDS. Even though the prognosis was worse, at least they were dealing with certainty.

Stress among Persons with AIDS

A diagnosis of AIDS is associated with multiple stressors. Health changes include new opportunistic infections and possible hospitalizations. These changes may interfere with job performance and relationships, causing further stress.

Eventually, job loss and the loss of income and health insurance may add to the level of distress. Some individuals find the loss of independence particularly difficult.

AIDS treatment is stressful. Clients must make difficult choices about taking multiple medications with potentially severe side effects. Participation in experimental drug protocols brings the added uncertainty of not knowing what to expect, either from treatment or side effects, or whether one is receiving only a placebo.

An additional problem associated with AIDS is that the physiological alterations caused by the virus and/or the drugs used to treat the disease may impair brain functioning. The person's perception, memory and problem-solving ability and, therefore, the ability to cope may be altered. (See Chapter 9, "Neuropsychological Functioning in HIV Disease.")

Stress Management Interventions

Stress reactions may impede individuals from participating in screening and early detection programs, impair acquisition of knowledge and skills necessary for prevention, foster treatment resistance and nonadherence, and result in negative health outcomes. Programs and interventions that include anticipation and reduction or management of distress hold tremendous potential for slowing the progression of HIV.

We cannot eliminate stress from our lives, but we can try to reduce it and to cope with it. We may change our life-style to reduce demands and increase fun. We can learn skills to improve our ability to respond to stressors.

Handling life stress successfully often calls for several abilities. The ability to accurately assess the stressful situation is important. The ability to relax quickly is also important. Finally, the ability to calmly do what is needed is useful. Stress management interventions may include training in any or all of these skills: relaxation, rational appraisal of events, and problem solving.

Stress Management Interventions

- Relaxation
- Cognitive restructuring
- Social support
- Exercise

To determine the best intervention, it is helpful first to determine the individual's usual response strategies through the course of their lifetime. Interventions should be aimed at enhancing and supplementing these strategies rather than simply replacing them. Coping strategies may include emotion-focused approaches, problem-focused approaches, seeking social support, and withdrawal or avoidance. Emotion-focused coping involves efforts aimed at reducing feelings of distress and physiological arousal, through activities such as relaxation or exercise. Problem-focused coping involves the individual's efforts to deal with the source of stress through behavior change or change in environmental conditions. Different strategies may be appropriate for different stressors.

Relaxation Training Techniques

Stress responses are often characterized by sympathetic CNS activation. Affective responses (e.g., anxiety) often accompany these responses, manifested in physical symptoms. Various types of relaxation training techniques have been developed to bring about states of psychological and physiological relaxation. These techniques have been used in treating a variety of physical problems including headache, hypertension, peptic ulcer disease, and pain, among others. Positive immunological changes have also been found in the use of these techniques.

Several types of relaxation procedures are used, including progressive muscle relaxation, deep muscle relaxation, transcendental meditation, autogenic training, and biofeedback. The various methods of relaxation training share several common features: (1) an emphasis on relaxation of particular sequences of muscle groups; (2) an emphasis on passive attention, or the opposite of striving or effort; and (3) encouragement to practice relaxation in everyday stressful situations. Relaxation skills can be taught in individual or group settings or can be learned, independently, using audio tapes.

Muscle relaxation techniques offer a way to control tension. The physical relaxation produced is pleasant and tends to leave the individual with a sense of refreshment. It is recommended that they be practiced twice a day for 15–30 minutes to achieve optimum benefit.

To progressively relax muscles, one begins by alternately tensing and relaxing the major muscle groups of the body. This helps to increase awareness of the body's muscular response to stress and of the difference between being tense and being relaxed. Tension accumulates in different muscles in different people and each individual can identify the specific areas where tension is troublesome. With continued practice, a person can achieve total relaxation throughout the body.

Deep muscle relaxation is similar to progressive relaxation but does not include the tensing part of the exercise. Instead, suggestions of relaxation are directed to each muscle group in turn. The individual learns to rely more on mental awareness, deep breathing, and calming words or phrases.

Relaxation is often combined with other behavioral and cognitive techniques to achieve optimum stress reduction benefits. Meditation techniques from a variety of cultures may be used. These usually include training in focused attention and increased ability to discriminate among feelings and perceptions. Systematic desensitization may also be used to replace unpleasant responses to stressors with newly learned relaxed responses.

Cognitive Restructuring

Although we usually think of events as being stressful, it is important to remember that the same event may be interpreted differently by different people. It is these interpretations that cause the stress reactions rather than the events themselves.

Because stress may be viewed as a result of cognitive appraisals that are based on a lack of information, misperception, or irrational beliefs, methods have been developed to assist individuals in changing their thought patterns. The same environmental challenges do not result in the same psychological or physiological changes in all individuals. Different persons will interpret the same circumstance differently. Cognitive restructuring is a process by which stress-provoking thoughts or beliefs are replaced with more constructive or realistic ones that reduce threat or harm appraisals. Ellis's Rational Emotive Therapy (RET) and Beck's cognitive therapy are two cognitive restructuring approaches.

With these approaches, an individual learns to identify the irrational or unhealthy beliefs that lead to feelings of distress. These often include exaggeration of the severity or consequences of a problem or minimizing one's ability to cope.

These strategies to improve coping may be applied with HIV-infected individuals. The next list shows some examples of irrational thoughts a person might have. Alternative thoughts that the individual might have, or that the clinician might suggest, are listed in italics.

"It's hopeless; I'm going to die."

"Everyone is going to die. I'm not going to die right now."

"Everyone I know will abandon me."

"Some people may abandon me, but I can find new support systems."

"I'm totally helpless; there's nothing I can do to affect the progress of the disease."

"I can take medicine and change my life-style to improve my condition."

"I won't be able to stand the pain."

"I can get medication to control the pain."

Enhancing Social Support

Social support is not only helpful after stressors appear, but it can also help avert the onset of problems. Adults can enhance their ability to give and receive social support by joining community organizations such as social, service, special interest, and self-help groups. Social skills training may be helpful for some individuals.

Especially important in health-related coping is the therapeutic use of support groups. Work with cancer patients has demonstrated that members of such groups model effective coping techniques, provide instrumental support, counter isolation, assist in pain control, and, perhaps, extend longevity (Fawzy et al., 1993; Spiegal, Bloom, and Yalom, 1981).

Because there is still stigma associated with HIV/AIDS, some infected people may find their previous support network disrupted as their condition becomes known. In this case, the individual should be encouraged to expand his or her network to include people who will provide support.

Importance of Physical Exercise

Exercise has been shown to both decrease distress and enhance physiological functioning. Recent studies of the effects of exercise on immune functioning show positive effects on both the number and the functioning of important immune cells. One study has shown aerobic exercise to act as a buffer to the affective distress that accompanies notification of HIV infection (La Perriere et al., 1990). In this study, aerobic exercise training was offered to individuals awaiting HIV test results. Of those who were found to be seropositive, the nonexercisers showed significant increases in anxiety and depression following notification while the exercisers showed no similar changes and, in fact, resembled those who received negative results.

Conclusion

In implementing any stress management intervention, the important thing to remember is that the goal is for the person to feel good. Even relaxation and exercise may be counterproductive if the individual becomes driven to perform the activity and feels guilty about omissions. Health benefits have been reported from a large range of activities including massage, listening to music, taking naps, and watching fish in a tank. The key is to increase the opportunities to experience pleasure and enjoy life. Of all the interventions designed to improve health, these may be the easiest to implement but the most likely to be overlooked.

Review Questions

1. The central nervous system and the immune system are interrelated. Describe a way in which each affects the other.

2. What are some significant life events that are likely to be associated with HIV/AIDS?

3. Describe three coping techniques to reduce stress.

Acknowledgments: The author wishes to express sincere thanks to Sally Dodds of the University of Miami Bio-psychosocial Learning Center on AIDS for her valuable contribution to this chapter.

References and Suggested Readings

Antoni, M.H., Schneiderman, N., Esterling, B., & Ironson, G. (1994). Stress management and adjustment to HIV-1 infection. *Homeostasis in Health and Disease, 35*(3), 149–160.

Blaney, N., Millon, C., Morgan, R., Eisdorfer, C., & Szapocznik, J. (1990). Emotional distress, stress-related disruption and coping among healthy HIV-1 positive gay males. *Psychology and Health, 4*(3), 259–273.

Blaney, N., Goodkin, K., Morgan, R., Feaster, D., Millon, C., & Szapocznik, J. (1991). A stress-moderator model of distress in early HIV-1 infection: Concurrent analyses of life events, hardiness, and social support. *Journal of Psychosomatic Research, 35*(2–3), 297–305.

Calabrese, J.R., Kling, M.A., & Gold, P.W. (1987). Alterations in immunocompetence during stress, bereavement and depression: Focus on neuroendocrine regulation. *American Journal of Psychiatry, 144*(a) 1123–1134.

Cohen, S. (1988). Voodoo death, the stress response, and AIDS. In T. Bridge, A. Mirsky, & F. Goodwin (Eds.), *Psychological, Neuropsychiatric and Substance Abuse Aspects of AIDS.* (95–109). New York: Raven Press.

Cohen, S., & Blumenthal, S. (1991). Psychoneuroimmunology and AIDS. In T. Janisse (Ed.), *Pain Management of AIDS Patients* (15–35). Boston: Kluwer Academic Publishers.

Cohen, S., & Williamson, G.M. (1991). Stress and infectious disease in humans. *Psychological Bulletin, 109*(1), 5–24.

Ellis, A. (1987). The impossibility of achieving consistently good mental health. *American Psychologist, 2,* 364–375.

Evans, D.L., Leserman, J., Perkins, D.O., & Stern, R.A. (1995). Stress-associated reductions of cytotoxic T lymphocytes and natural killer cells in asymptomatic HIV infection. *American Journal of Psychiatry, 152*(4), 543–550.

Fawzy, F.I., Fawzy, N.W., Hyun, C.S., Elashoff, R., Guthrie, D., Fahey, J.L., & Morton, D.L. (1993). Malignant melanoma: Effects of an early structured psychiatric intervention, coping, and affective state on recurrence and survival 6 years later. *Archives of General Psychiatry, 50,* 681–689.

Glaser, R., & Kiecolt-Glaser, J.K. (Eds.) (1994). *Handbook of Human Stress and Immunity.* San Diego: Academic Press.

Gorman, J.M., & Kertzner, R.M. (Eds.) (1991). *Psychoimmunology Update.* Washington, D.C.: American Psychiatric Press.

Huggins, J., Elman, N., Baker, C., Forrester, R., & Lyter, D. (1991). Affective and behavioral responses of gay and bisexual men to HIV antibody testing. *Social Work, 36*(1), 61–66.

Holmes, T.H., & Rahe, R.H. (1967). The Social Readjustment Rating Scale. *Journal of Psychosomatic Research, 11,* 213–218.

Kiecolt-Glaser, J., & Glaser, R. (1988). Psychological influences on immunity: Implications for AIDS. *American Psychologist, 43,* 892–898.

La Perriere, A., Antoni, M., Schneiderman, N., Ironson, G., Klimas, N., Caralis, P., & Fletcher, M. (1990). Exercise intervention attenuates emotional distress and natural killer cell decrements following notification of positive serologic status for HIV-1. *Biofeedback and Self-Regulation, 15*(3), 229–242.

Levy, S.M. (1985). *Behavior and Cancer.* San Francisco: Jossey-Bass.

Noh, S., Chandarana, P., Field, V., & Posthuma, B. (1990). AIDS epidemics, emotional strain, coping and psychological distress in homosexual men. *AIDS Education and Prevention, 2,* 272–283.

Nott, K.H., Vedhara, K., & Spickett, G.P. (1995). Psychology, immunology, and HIV. *Psychoneuroendocrinology, 20*(5), 451–474.

Ornstein, R., & Sobel, D. (1989). *Healthy Pleasures.* Woburn, MA: Addison-Wesley.

Perkins, D. (1982). The assessment of stress using life events scales. In S. Breznitz & L. Goldberger (Eds.), *Handbook of Stress: Theoretical and Clinical Aspects.* (320–331). New York: Free Press.

Rogers, M.P. (1989). The interaction between brain behavior and immunity. In S. Cheren (Ed.), *Psychosomatic Medicine: Theory, Physiology, and Practice.* (279–330). Madison, CT: International University Press.

Schneiderman, N., McCabe, P., & Baum, A. (1992). *Stress and Disease Processes.* Hillsdale, NJ: Lawrence Erlbaum Associates.

Siemens, H. (1993). A Gestalt approach in the care of persons with HIV. *Gestalt Journal, 16*(1), 91–104.

Spiegal, D., Bloom, J., & Yalom, I. (1981). Group support for patients with metastatic cancer: A randomized prospective outcome study. *Archives of General Psychiatry, 38*(5), 527–533.

Temoshok, L., Heller, B.W., Sagebiel, R.W., Blois, M.S., Sweet, D.M., DiClemente, R.J., & Gold, M.L. (1985). The relationship of psychosocial factors to prognostic indicators in cutaneous malignant melanoma. *Journal of Psychosomatic Research, 29,* 139–153.

Tross, S., & Hirsch, D. (1988). Psychological distress and neurological complications of HIV infection and AIDS. *American Psychologist, 43,* 929–934.

Weiner, H., Fawzy, I., & Fawzy, M.D. (1989). An integrative model of health, disease, and illness. In S. Cheren (Ed.), *Psychosomatic Medicine: Theory, Physiology, and Practice.* (9–45). Madison, CT: International University Press.

Chapter 12

Depression and HIV Disease

Michael G. Dow, Ph.D.

Overview

Depression is common among HIV-infected persons seen in community mental health centers (CMHCs). This chapter summarizes basic information about depression, theories of causation, diagnosis, and the relationships between HIV infection and depression. The role of cognitive distortion in maintaining high-risk behavior is discussed. Various treatment approaches are presented.

Learning Objectives

1. To identify symptoms that are common to depression and HIV infection.

2. To provide at least five examples of cognitive distortions that may increase the risk of HIV infection.

3. To specify at least two ways that the treatment of depression would be complicated by the presence of HIV infection.

Outline

I. The Relationship between HIV Infection and Depression

A. Basic information about depression
1. Prevalence
2. Diagnostic criteria

B. Theories of causation

C. Commonality of symptoms—identifying HIV infection among persons with depression
1. Relationships between HIV-induced medical conditions and depression
2. Depression versus dementia
3. Suicide risk
4. Transitions between anxiety and depression in persons with HIV disease
5. Depression and grieving among the family and friends of persons with HIV disease

II. Depression as a Risk Factor for Contracting HIV Infection

A. The role of cognitive distortion in maintaining high-risk behavior

B. The role of cognitive distortion among persons with HIV infection who risk giving the disease to others

C. Depression and substance abuse—risk factors for HIV infection

D. HIV infection and bipolar disorder

III. Treatment Approaches

A. HIV risk reduction among persons with depression

B. Cognitive-behavioral approaches

C. Self-monitoring of behavior

D. Targeting social interactions

E. Pharmacological interventions

IV. Conclusion

The Relationship between HIV Infection and Depression

Depression has been considered to be the "common cold" of psychological problems. Most people have felt somewhat "down" or depressed at various points in their lives, so most of us can understand the feelings of sadness and discouragement that depressed people experience. Clinical depression brings with it a variety of cognitive, behavioral, and physical symptoms, such as feelings of hopelessness, indecision, and inability to act. Collectively, these symptoms are experienced as more devastating than depressed mood alone. Persons who first experience clinical depression may not know that they are depressed and may state that they have no idea how they came to feel the way they do. They may believe that no one else has ever felt that way before.

Basic Information about Depression

Prevalence

Clinical depression is relatively common. Scientific studies show that approximately 5 percent of the adult population is clinically depressed at any one time (Dow, 1993). Depression is about twice as common in women as it is in men. In terms of lifetime prevalence, approximately 20 percent of all women experience a major affective disorder at some point in their lives, as compared with approximately 10 percent of all men.

Since depression is so common, some of the persons who acquire HIV infection, or who are at risk for HIV infection, may have been clinically depressed. Others with no history of depression may develop depression after learning that they are HIV-positive. Others may experience symptoms of HIV infection that are difficult to distinguish from symptoms of depression. It is sometimes difficult to unravel the ways in which depression and HIV disease may be related. This chapter attempts to clarify some of these interrelationships and to remind clinicians about these issues.

Diagnostic Criteria

Major Symptoms of Clinical Depression

- Depressed mood
- Lowered interest or pleasure in most activities
- Significant weight gain or weight loss when not dieting
- Insomnia or hypersomnia
- Psychomotor agitation or retardation
- Fatigue or loss of energy
- Feelings of worthlessness or guilt
- Lowered ability to think or concentrate, or indecisiveness
- Recurrent thoughts of death, suicidal ideations, or suicide attempt

■ Symptoms causing distress or impairment in functioning

■ Symptoms not resulting from the physiological effects of a substance or a general medical condition

■ Disturbance not a situational grief reaction

Based on *DSM-IV* (American Psychiatric Association, 1994)

The list shows the major symptoms of clinical depression. At least five of the symptoms must be evident nearly every day for more than two weeks to be considered significant for a diagnosis of depression. One of the symptoms must be depressed mood or loss of interest or pleasure. People who also have manic episodes may be diagnosed with bipolar disorder. Persons who experience a fairly chronic form of mild depression over a two-year period, without meeting the full criteria for major depressive disorder, may be diagnosed with dysthymic disorder. Persons who experience depressed mood after a specific event, or a series of events, but do not meet the criteria for major depressive disorder, may be diagnosed with adjustment disorder with depressed mood. This type of depression must occur within three months of the stressful event and not persist longer than six months after the precipitating event ends.

Theories of Causation

There have been several theories of depression, all of which may have some value in explaining the constellation of symptoms called depression. This next list shows five major theories.

Theories of Depression

■ Psychodynamic

■ Behavioral

■ Cognitive

■ Biological

■ Humanistic/existential

The psychodynamic approach refers to depression as anger turned inward, as well as the experience of a lost love object. Early childhood loss experiences are supposed to predispose people to experience depression later in life during times of loss or frustration.

The behavioral approach to depression emphasizes reduced positive reinforcement. According to Peter Lewinsohn and others, this is often due to reduced social skill, fewer opportunities for reinforcement, and other environmental constraints, such as the loss of a loved one who provided reinforcement (Lewinsohn and Hoberman, 1982). An individual who is not reinforced for attempts to engage others in social relationships may become depressed. Some behaviorists emphasize the cognitive process of making attributions about events, in addition to the events themselves.

Some authors, such as Aaron Beck (1967), emphasize the cognitive aspects of depression. People become depressed largely as a result of cognitive bias or cognitive distortion of events. This cognitive style may be formed from early loss experiences, but becomes the primary factor.

Depressed persons may be predisposed to a negative view of themselves, the world, and the future. A depressed person engages in a series of cognitive errors such as arbitrarily inferring motives or meaning from events, maximizing the impact of negative events and minimizing the impact of positive events, personalizing, and overgeneralizing.

The biological approach emphasizes reduced rates of brain neurotransmitters, particularly norepinephrine and serotonin. While emphasizing a biological predisposition to depression and pharmacological treatment, this theory, as usually expressed, does allow for the role of environmental events and stress in further reducing the availability of brain neurotransmitters.

The humanistic approach emphasizes the individual's unique phenomenological position as an organism who observes himself or herself and looks for meaning and purpose in life. When an individual is frustrated in the development of personal growth, depression may set in. The experience of death, disease, and other problems challenges the individual's ability to see meaning and purpose. If unable to alleviate these concerns, they can overwhelm an individual, producing depression, alienation of self, and alienation from others.

All of these models seem to shed some light on the development of depression. They are not necessarily incompatible with each other, although they tend to differ in degree of emphasis placed on certain routes to depression.

Several of the theoretical issues just discussed may have some relevance to HIV infection. The HIV-positive person who experienced significant loss as a child may be more likely to reexperience those losses and become depressed as an adult, according to the psychodynamic viewpoint. An HIV-positive person who has lost relationships, become socially isolated, and failed to break out of the pattern of reduced positive reinforcement that this brings may be more likely to be depressed, according to the behavioral position. Cognitive distortions and cognitive errors are crucial in the cognitive position. Basic biology may be relevant as well, providing a predisposition to depression. The way the HIV-positive person views his or her life and society as a whole may be influential, according to the humanistic position.

A recent study on men with hemophilia indicated that HIV-positive men were more likely to be depressed than those who were not HIV-positive (Dew, Ragni, and Nimorwicz, 1990). Characteristics of the HIV-positive persons which were most influential in determining level of depression included the following: personal history of mental illness, family history of mental illness, relatively low educational level, low social support, reduced sense of personal mastery, and recent loss experiences.

George Brown and colleagues (Brown et al., 1992) researched the prevalence of psychological disorders among a large group of men screened for HIV by the military. They found that, although the HIV-positive individuals were more likely to be depressed than were age-matched controls in the general population, part of this difference was a result of a higher rate of mood and substance use disorders before HIV screening.

Finally, Kelly et al. (1993) assessed a large group of HIV-infected men and found that individuals who became HIV-infected had low social support, were likely to believe that health was influenced by chance, and had engaged in high-risk sexual behavior.

Commonality of Symptoms—Identifying HIV Infection among Persons with Depression

Some of the physical symptoms of HIV infection are the same, or similar, to the symptoms of depression. These include weight loss, decreased appetite, somatic concerns such as headaches and pain, irritability, tiredness, lethargy, sleep difficulties (possibly brought on by night sweats or fever), and problems with thinking, memory, or concentration. These symptoms are shown in the next list.

Common Symptoms of Depression and HIV Infection

- Weight loss
- Decreased appetite
- Somatic concerns—headache, pain, etc.
- Irritability
- Tiredness
- Lethargy
- Sleep difficulties
- Problems with thinking, memory, or concentration

The individual may also respond to news of being HIV-positive with an emotional reaction such as anger, sadness, discouragement, or a sense of hopelessness. Most persons who become depressed after learning of HIV infection can be presumed to be experiencing a "reactive" depression.

Relationships between HIV-Induced Medical Conditions and Depression

Research by Gorman et al. (1991) indicated that HIV-positive persons with the greatest degree of medical complications were also most likely to be depressed and anxious. The direction of causation may well be twofold, as a number of authors have speculated that stress-induced activation of the hypothalamic-pituitary-adrenal (HPA) axis may tend to compromise the immune system and increase symptoms of HIV infection. The data do not yet appear conclusive in this area of study. Fernandez and Levy (1994) cautioned about the importance of identifying and treating all physical symptoms of HIV infection. It should not be assumed that any physical problem is caused only by depression. Examples include: anemia, myopathy, gastritis, disturbances of metabolism, diarrhea, and multifocal leukoencephalopathy.

Lyketsos et al. (1996) investigated the course of depressive symptoms among HIV-positive persons. They found that two to five years before AIDS developed, depressive symptoms were stable. However, beginning eighteen months before the diagnosis of AIDS, there was a significant increase in all measures of depression, reaching a fairly stable level for the last six months before full-blown AIDS.

Persons who are HIV-infected may experience stressors including: less physical activity, reduced social life, guilt, ruminating thoughts, and confronting death. These are some of the reasons why a person may experience depression as the physical symptoms of HIV disease increase. As warning signs, they may indicate the need for early intervention on the part of caregivers and counselors.

As one becomes physically ill from HIV infection, one may become less mobile and more restricted in one's activities, reducing opportunities for positive reinforcement. Some friends, acquaintances, and relatives may abandon the HIV-infected person, further reducing opportunities for reinforcement and setting up a situation where negative self-labeling, guilt, and negative thoughts can magnify the depression. The experience of confronting one's own death may raise existential concerns, including thoughts about one's accomplishments, regrets about past actions, and confusion about the human condition. All of these factors may make it more difficult to treat depression in persons with HIV infection.

Depression versus Dementia

Another type of medical condition that sometimes accompanies HIV infection, especially in the later stages of the disorder, is dementia. The effort to distinguish depression and dementia is another concern. While it is common for depressed individuals to have some mental slowing, some memory problems, and some confusion, these symptoms seem to vary with the experience of depression and show fairly quick rebound as the person recovers from depression. Many cognitive difficulties of a depressed person stem from attention problems—difficulty encoding and processing information because of ruminative thinking. With dementia, such as might be brought on by HIV infection, performance of specific functions is more consistently impoverished and tends not to show as much recovery.

Suicide Risk

Suicidal ideation, thoughts of death, and suicidal behavior, including suicide attempts, are fairly common symptoms of depression. Research has shown that males are more likely to actually take their own lives, while females make more attempts (Rich, Ricketts, Fowler, and Young, 1988). Men who are not involved in intimate relationships, are over 50, and live alone are among those most likely to kill themselves. People with an agitated form of depression, which includes some anxiety, may also be likelier to kill themselves. Relief from ruminative thinking—constant negative thinking and preoccupation—is often one of the more immediate goals of suicide. A manipulative attempt to control others, a cry for help, and an effort to control one's life by managing one's death are other theories of causation.

One study by Marzuk et al. (1988) showed that gay men diagnosed with AIDS in New York City were 36 times more likely to commit suicide than men who did not have AIDS. Other research has shown that persons with HIV infection may be somewhat more likely to attempt suicide before the development of full-blown AIDS, rather than after the full range of symptoms develop. The diagnosis of AIDS may bring some cessation to the mental torment of "what's going to happen to me?" (See Chapter 11, "Stress Effects: The Relationship Between Health and Stress.") The opportunity for adjustment to the situation and resignation may bring with it reduced chance of suicide.

Transitions between Anxiety and Depression in Persons with HIV Disease

One of the key similarities between depression and anxiety is the expectation of negative outcomes. However, a depressed person often feels unable to control the situation and expects a negative outcome, while an anxious person still has a sense of personal control, and, therefore, responsibility to continue to try to prevent the negative outcome. Much of the pressure felt by anxious persons comes from the continued activation of their "fight or flight response." A depressed person has given up and is relatively confident that negative events will occur, while an anxious person senses less predictability. With HIV infection, the individual may move back and forth between the sense of personal control, unpredictability, and agitation, versus helplessness, prediction of negative outcome, and despair. Anxiety may better characterize the first phase; depression, the second phase.

Depression and Grieving among the Family and Friends of
Persons with HIV Disease

The circumstances of HIV infection, if known or believed to be known, may influence the grief reaction of family and friends. The timeliness with which information about the infection is disseminated to friends and loved ones may also be important. (See Chapter 10, "Notifying Others of Seropositivity.") In some instances, parents first learn that a son is HIV-positive at the same time they first learn that he is gay or an injecting drug user. This may bring about a dual sense of loss.

Grief often involves a sense of guilt. People often ask questions such as: "Could I have done more to be a good parent? Could I have prevented this?" Parents are not prepared to outlive their children. The sense of disorder this brings adds to the sense of unfairness and despair.

The impact of HIV infection on the gay community has been widely documented. While the gay community has rallied to offer social support and acceptance, incidents of prejudice and discrimination from the broader community have increased.

Depression as a Risk Factor for Contracting HIV Infection

The Role of Cognitive Distortion in Maintaining High-Risk Behaviors

After the release of the Surgeon General's report (U.S. Public Health Service, 1964) that concluded that smoking was dangerous, the proportion of smokers in the United States gradually declined for approximately 10 years or more, but then the rate of smoking seemed to stabilize (Surgeon General, 1979). This demonstrates that compelling evidence does not always result in behavior that promotes self-preservation. The process of ignoring important information and maintaining high-risk behavior is a process that could be described as cognitive distortion. Just as some depressed persons distort information about their own personal adequacy and focus on evidence of incompetence, many people continue to engage in high-risk behavior for HIV infection, despite adequate knowledge of the danger.

The next list outlines several examples of cognitive distortions that increase a person's risk of contracting HIV disease.

Cognitions That May Help Maintain High-Risk Behaviors for HIV Infection

- Everyone is going to die of something anyway.
- Life isn't worth living without sex (or injecting drugs).
- I don't expect to live a long time anyway.
- By the time I catch it, they'll have a cure.
- Only hookers and people who are really promiscuous get it.
- I couldn't talk to someone about using a condom, so I'll just have to trust my partner.
- Chances are that I won't get it.
- I might already be infected so it's too late now.

The Role of Cognitive Distortion among Persons with HIV Infection Who Risk Giving the Disease to Others

One of the more difficult clinical situations that a case manager or therapist may encounter occurs when an HIV-positive client talks about having unprotected sex or sharing injection drug paraphernalia with another person. Whether there is a "duty to warn" the other person in this situation is something that should be considered aggressively by the mental health field and by individual therapists. The type of rationalization that the client must be engaged in to continue risking the health and life of another person is certainly important material for therapy. In the effort to help the therapist identify and challenge these assumptions, the next list provides several examples of cognitive distortions that might make an HIV-positive person more likely to risk infecting others.

Cognitions That Might Make an HIV-Positive Person More Likely to Risk Giving the Infection to Others

- I don't have any symptoms, so maybe I don't really have AIDS.
- It's up to my partner to protect himself or herself.
- I deserve to have some enjoyment before I get sick.
- This person might be infected already.
- I'm not responsible for anyone but myself.

■ If I insist on using a condom, my partner might think I'm infected and leave.

■ It will be OK as long as we don't have . . . (anal intercourse, vaginal intercourse, etc.).

Depression and Substance Abuse—Risk Factors for HIV Infection

Alcohol and many other drugs have disinhibiting effects on behavior. Thus, an individual may be more likely to engage in high-risk behavior when engaged in substance use and abuse. Research has shown that depressed persons are somewhat more likely to abuse drugs and alcohol. Thus, these dually diagnosed persons deserve some special mention. Ekstrand and Coates (1990) examined gay men who resumed having unprotected anal intercourse following previous precautionary changes in sexual behavior. They found that substance abuse was one of the major predictors of relapse into high-risk behavior. Brown et al. (1992) found higher rates of substance abuse among HIV-infected military recruits, compared with rates of age-matched controls. (See Chapter 18, "Treating Persons Who Use Drugs.")

HIV Infection and Bipolar Disorder

Individuals with bipolar disorder often act out in impulsive ways when experiencing a manic episode. A sense of invulnerability and grandiosity is often present, which keeps an individual from recognizing real risks. Substance abuse and sexual activity are often associated with manic episodes, further compounding these problems.

Treatment Approaches

There are a number of treatment issues that could be emphasized in considering the relationship between HIV disease and depression. One issue is that there may be reason to believe that HIV risk reduction could be somewhat more difficult in some individuals who are depressed.

HIV Risk Reduction among Persons with Depression

When a person is depressed, he or she may not take usual, proper precautions to ensure his or her own safety. The concept of a passive suicidal gesture is based on this idea. The man who is upset and drives fast risks his own life but may not be actively or consciously attempting suicide. So too, the depressed person who risks HIV infection may be influenced by depressive thinking. Attempts to straightforwardly tell depressed persons how they should act to preserve their health and safety may not work. Depressed persons also tend not to be appropriately assertive. Having a negative view of oneself may make it more difficult to turn down unwanted sexual advances, to require a sexual partner to use a condom, or to insist that needles be washed in bleach or not shared. For these reasons, a special emphasis on HIV risk reduction seems appropriate with depressed persons.

However, there are also some reasons to consider depression to be a protective factor in reducing risk of HIV infection in some people. Depression brings greater social isolation, which could reduce the risk of infection. Depressed persons may also have reduced interest in sex. One study by Kelly, St. Lawrence, and Brasfield (1991) found that resumption of certain high-risk behavior by gay men was more likely among individuals with a low score on a depression measure. Although depression may decrease the risk of HIV infection in some people, it may increase the risk in others.

Cognitive-Behavioral Approaches

Many of the cognitive-behavioral approaches to depression may be effective with persons who are depressed and have HIV infection. The basic cognitive therapy approach can be simplified as shown in the next list. The overall goal is to help the client see that, although his or her depression may be caused by major issues such as HIV infection, there are day-to-day negative experiences and negative thoughts that maintain the depression. Dealing with these maintaining issues is often helpful in reducing depressed mood and ultimately reducing the depression.

Changing Depressive Thinking

Describe a specific recent situation that brought out your feelings of depression.

I met someone who seemed nice, and as we were talking I realized he had a cold. I started worrying about getting sick.

List your negative self-statements that made the depression feel worse.

If I catch his cold, I might die. There's no reason to talk to him; if he knew I was HIV-positive, he'd run away. Life is not worth living. I was such a fool to have unprotected sex with many partners. My life is over. I never should have been born. I am a failure.

Argue against those negative self-statements.

I can choose to continue talking to him or go away. I am still in control of my life. It doesn't help me to think negative thoughts, so I am going to shut off these negative ideas. The past is past, I am going to live for now.

List some positive self-statements.

I still have a lot to offer others. I can help make others aware of AIDS and work for positive social change. Many people live for years after becoming HIV-positive. I will face my situation and live the best life I can. I am somebody.

The above are examples of how a person with HIV infection and depression might think in a typically depressed way. An incident occurs, and a spiral of negative thinking follows. A person who has been trained in cognitive therapy techniques should be able to stop an onslaught of negative thinking before it drives the person down into a very low mood.

Self-Monitoring of Behavior

Research has shown that attempts to reduce smoking, reduce weight, or increase positive activities are often helped by careful self-monitoring of behavior (Nelson and Hayes, 1981). When forced to account for our behavior, in writing, we are often motivated to behave in the ways that are socially acceptable or desired. A time clock does wonders for helping employees get to work on time, for example. There are several ways that self-monitoring can be employed by persons with HIV disease. First, one of the standard treatments for depression, developed by Lewinsohn and colleagues, involves identifying potentially important positive behavior, recording the daily frequency of that behavior, and attempting to systematically increase positive events (Lewinshon and Hoberman, 1982). The same type of approach can be used to record instances of HIV risk behaviors. Depending on the needs of clients, you could ask them to record aspects of their sexual behavior, such as the number of sexual partners they have, and whether or not condoms were used, or you could record information about injection drug usage and precautions taken.

Targeting Social Interactions

Depressed persons often avoid social situations, which limits their opportunities for pleasurable events, and may compound their depression. Depressed persons also appear less socially skilled in introductory conversations. The treatment approach usually recommended is to work with depressed persons to gradually increase the number of social situations they are involved in and to enhance their social skill level. Efforts to increase social activities may be more difficult, however, because of the medical problems and reduced social and familial support that sometimes is associated with HIV infection. Efforts to improve social skills may include assertiveness training and role-playing of practice conversations. Helping clients to negotiate sexual behavior and the use of condoms may be particularly important.

Pharmacological Interventions

Research on depressed persons has shown that the combination of cognitive-behavioral therapy and antidepressant medication is often more effective than either type of treatment alone. If only one type of treatment is used, most researchers seem to have concluded that cognitive-behavioral approaches are comparable in effectiveness to antidepressant medications and may be somewhat easier to tolerate.

As discussed by Harnett (1994), physicians may tend not to medicate depressed HIV-positive individuals as aggressively as other depressed patients. The belief that such depression is reactive to a difficult life event may be part of the reason, as is the finding, at least in rodents, that antidepressants may induce worsening of immune status (Brandes, Arron, and Bogdarovic, 1992). Antidepressant medications also often have significant side effects, which may be more difficult to tolerate in individuals already experiencing physical symptoms. Some of the common antidepressant side effects overlap with symptoms of HIV infection and may include dizziness, weakness, nausea, headaches, sweating, and insomnia (Harnett, 1994). Despite these concerns, imipramine was superior to placebo in a double-blind controlled study on depressed HIV-infected patients (Rabkin, Rabkin, Harrison, and Wagner, 1994). Psychostimulants, such as methylphenidate, may also be helpful in some cases and may reduce HIV-related cognitive impairment (Harnett, 1994). One study (Wagner, Rabkin, and Rabkin, 1996) compared traditional antidepressants (imipramine, fluoxetine, and sertraline) with alternative drugs (dextroamphetamine and testosterone) in the treatment of depressed HIV-positive patients. Response rates were similar and both better than placebo. A final concern, discussed by Fernandez and Levy (1994), is the possibility that antidepressants may interact adversely with antiviral or other medical treatments. Based on evidence, despite several areas of concern, it does appear that antidepressant medications are often helpful in the comprehensive treatment of depression among HIV-positive individuals. Medical consultation seems to be an important part of a comprehensive evaluation of depression, from both an assessment and treatment perspective. Some specific guidelines related to the use of fluoxetine, nortriptyline, desipramine, and sertraline with individuals experiencing infectious disease are found on page 223 of the book by Bartlett (1996).

Conclusion

Depression is a fairly frequent occurrence among HIV-infected persons. Several of the symptoms of HIV infection are also symptoms of depression. Thus, CMHC staff need to be aware of these joint symptoms, carefully diagnose these conditions, and provide appropriate treatments. Many of the theoretical formulations and treatment strategies used with depression are also relevant if the depressed person has HIV infection. The model of cognitive distortion that is discussed in this area may also be informative when thinking about the process an individual goes through to maintain high-risk behavior for HIV infection or to risk giving the infection to others. Therapeutic approaches that help the individual examine these thoughts, test the rationality of the thoughts, and exhibit behavior that is more consistent with long-range personal goals and socially responsible behavior are applicable. The use of antidepressant medications is often helpful, although some individuals find it difficult to tolerate the side effects.

Review Questions

1. Identify three common symptoms of depressed mood.

2. What might lead a person to justify unprotected sexual practices?

3. Name two reasons that a person who is HIV-positive might be mistakenly diagnosed as depressed by an intake worker.

4. What is a cognitive-behavioral treatment of depression?

References and Suggested Readings

American Psychiatric Association. (1994). *Diagnostic and Statistical Manual of Mental Disorders* (4th ed.). Washington, D.C.

Bartlett, J.G. (1996). *Pocket Book of Infectious Disease Therapy.* Baltimore: Williams & Wilkins.

Beck, A.T. (1967). *Depression: Causes and Treatment.* Philadelphia: University of Pennsylvania Press.

Blackburn, I.M., Bishop, S., Glen, A.I.M., Whalley, L.J., & Christie, J.E. (1981). The efficacy of cognitive therapy in depression: A treatment trial using cognitive therapy and pharmacotherapy, each alone and in combination. *British Journal of Psychiatry, 139,* 181–189.

Brandes, L.J., Arron, R.J., & Bogdarovic, R.P. (1992). Stimulation of malignant growth in rodents by antidepressant drugs at clinically relevant doses. *Cancer Research, 52,* 3796–3800.

Brown, G.R., Rundell, J.R., McManis, S.E., Kendall, S.N., Zachary, R., & Temoshok, L. (1992). Prevalence of psychiatric disorders in early stages of HIV infection. *Psychosomatic Medicine, 54,* 588–601.

Dew, M.A., Ragni, M.V., & Nimorwicz, P. (1990). Infection with human immunodeficiency virus and vulnerability to psychiatric distress. *Archives of General Psychiatry, 47,* 737–744.

Dow, M.G. (1993). Affective disorders. In A.S. Bellack & M. Hersen (Eds.), *Handbook of Behavior Therapy in the Psychiatric Setting.* (251–268). New York: Plenum.

Ekstrand, M.L., & Coates, T.J. (1990). Maintenance of safer sexual behaviors and predictors of risky sex: The San Francisco men's health study. *American Journal of Public Health, 80,* 973–977.

Fernandez, F., & Levy, J.K. (1994). Psychopharmacology in HIV spectrum disorders. *Psychiatric Clinics of North America, 17,* 135–148.

Gorman, J.M., Kertzner, R., Cooper, T., Goetz, R.R., Lagomasino, I., Novacenko, H., Williams, J.B.W., Stern, Y., Mayeux, R., & Ehrhardt, A.A. (1991). Glucocorticoid level and neuropsychiatric symptoms in homosexual men with HIV infection. *American Journal of Psychiatry, 148,* 41–45.

Harnett, D.S. (1994). Psychopharmacologic treatment of depression in the medical setting. *Psychiatric Annals, 24,* 545–551.

Hays, R.B., Turner, H., & Coates, T.J. (1992). Social support, AIDS-related symptoms, and depression among gay men. *Journal of Consulting and Clinical Psychology, 60,* 463–469.

Holland, J.C., & Tross, S. (1985). The psychosocial and neuropsychiatric sequelae of the acquired immunodeficiency syndrome and related disorders. *Annals of Internal Medicine, 103,* 760–764.

Kelly, J.A., St. Lawrence, J.S., & Brasfield, T.L. (1991). Predictors of vulnerability to AIDS risk behavior relapse. *Journal of Consulting and Clinical Psychology, 59,* 163–166.

Kelly, J.A., Murphy, D.A., Bahr, G.R., Koob, J.J., Morgan, M.G., Kalichman, S.C., Stevenson, L.Y., Brasfield, T.L., Bernstein, B.M., & St. Lawrence, J.S. (1993). Factors associated with severity of depression and high risk sexual behavior among persons diagnosed with HIV infection. *Health Psychology, 12,* 215–219.

Lewinsohn, P.M., & Hoberman, H.M. (1982). Behavioral and cognitive approaches. In E.S. Paykel (Ed.), *Handbook of Affective Disorders.* New York: Guilford Press.

Lyketsos, C.G., Hoover, D.R., Guccione, M., Dew, M.A., Wesch, J.E., Bing, E.G., & Treisman, G.T. (1996). Changes in depressive symptoms as AIDS develops. *American Journal of Psychiatry, 153,* 1430–1437.

Marzuk, P., Tierney, H., Tardiff, K., Gross, E., Morgan, E., Hsu, M., & Mann, J. (1988). Increased risk of suicide in persons with AIDS. *Journal of the American Medical Association, 259,* 1333–1337.

Nelson, R.O., & Hayes, S.C. (1981). Theoretical explanations for reactivity in self-monitoring. *Behavior Modification, 5,* 3–14.

Perry, S.W., & Tross, S. (1984). Psychiatric problems of AIDS inpatients at the New York Hospital: Preliminary report. *Public Health Reports, 99,* 200–205.

Rabkin, J.G., Rabkin, R., Harrison, W., & Wagner, G. (1994). Effect of imipramine on mood and enumerative measures of immune status in depressed patients with HIV illness. *American Journal of Psychiatry, 151,* 516–523.

Rich, C.L., Ricketts, J.E., Fowler, R.C., & Young, D. (1988). Some differences between men and women who commit suicide. *American Journal of Psychiatry, 145,* 718–722.

Surgeon General. (1979). Modification of smoking behavior. In *Smoking and Health: A Report of the Surgeon General.* Washington D.C.: U.S. Department of Health and Human Services Publication (PHS) 79-50066.

U.S. Public Health Service. (1964). *Smoking and Health: Report of the Advisory Committee to the Surgeon General of the Public Health Service* (U.S. Public Health Service Publication No. 1103). Washington, D.C.: U.S. Government Printing Office.

Wagner, G., Rabkin, J.G., & Rabkin, R.. (1996). A comparative analysis of standard and alternative antidepressants in the treatment of human immunodeficiency virus patients. *Comprehensive Psychiatry, 37,* 402–408.

Chapter 13

■ Suicide Assessment and Intervention
with Persons Infected with HIV

Mary Kay Houston-Vega, Ph.D., M.S.W.,
and John C. Ward, Jr., Ph.D.

Overview

This chapter addresses the important issues of assessing suicidal risk and planning effective interventions with persons infected with HIV. The text is written with the assumption that the reader will have gained some requisite knowledge and skills from other chapters in this book, specifically those on depression, preparing for death, and neuropsychological functioning in HIV disease. Sections of the chapter were adapted from the *Screener's Handbook for Mental Health Emergency Intervention* (1988) by Mary Kay Houston and Elane Nuehring.

Learning Objectives

1. To demonstrate familiarity with the characteristics of persons infected with HIV who may be at risk for suicide.

2. To identify the phases of crisis intervention and suicide assessment, including specific questions to ask the client.

3. To describe how to mobilize supportive resources.

Outline

I. Overview of Potential Suicide
- A. Current research on HIV and suicide
- B. Risk factors and predictors related to HIV/AIDS
- C. Stages of HIV disease
  1. Psychological stages of HIV disease
  2. Characteristics of terminally ill persons who commit suicide

II. Crisis Intervention and Suicide Risk Assessment
- A. Identifying stressors and exploring a client's intent
  1. HIV-related stressors
  2. Suicide risk factors for HIV-infected gay men
  3. Questions to ask the client
  4. Verbal and behavioral predictors of suicidal behavior
- B. Exploring the seriousness of a suicide plan
  1. Availability
  2. Lethality
  3. Proximity
  4. Specificity
- C. Assessing coping skills
- D. Immediate versus long-term risks
- E. Suicide intervention

Overview of Potential Suicide

Mental health providers who help persons with HIV infection or AIDS must be ready to deal with a variety of complex situations. One of the most challenging and emotionally charged is the risk of suicide. People who are aware of their HIV infection or who face debilitating symptoms of opportunistic infection from AIDS often exhibit signs of depression, confusion and anger, and a sense of helplessness and hopelessness. The initial, and sometimes persistent, reaction to the awareness of any life-threatening disease can be loss of self-esteem, autonomy, and hope for a fulfilling life. If left unchecked and unchallenged, these reactions may lead to self-destructive thoughts and actions aimed at ending the physical and emotional distress.

Current Research on HIV and Suicide

For over a decade, clinicians have been aware of and concerned about identifying suicidal risk factors of persons with HIV infection. The findings are contradictory. In a study by McKegney and O'Dowd (1992), persons with AIDS had a significantly lower suicide rate than persons who were asymptomatic, and they did not appear to differ in suicide rates from persons with unknown or negative HIV status. Other studies report higher rates of suicide attempts and completions for persons with asymptomatic HIV infection and AIDS when compared with the general population (Cote, Biggar, and Dannenberg, 1992; Marzuk et al., 1988; Kizer et al., 1988; Mancoske, Wadsworth, Dugas, and Hasney, 1995). Other studies have determined that injecting drug users (IDUs) who are HIV-positive pose a greater risk of death by suicide and overdose when compared with IDUs who do not know their HIV status (van Haastrecht, Mientjes, van den Hoek, and Coutinho, 1994).

In 1993, O'Dowd, Biderman, and McKegney reported that persons with more advanced symptoms of AIDS had significantly fewer suicidal ideations than persons who were HIV-positive with few or no symptoms. They concluded that the lower rate of suicidality could be explained by these factors: the refocusing of life goals, denial, and the psychological impact of central nervous system impairment. van Haastrecht, Mientjes, van den Hoek, and Coutinho (1994) also reported that, for persons who were IDUs in Amsterdam, receiving an HIV-positive diagnosis did not contribute to an immediate increase in suicide.

Research findings are often difficult to compare because researchers report measures in ways that may not be comparable (e.g., attempts versus completions, or ideation versus attempts). Predictors of one may not reliably predict the other. Findings are also confounded by reports that suicides of persons with HIV or AIDS may be underreported or incorrectly reported as "death resulting from complications of HIV."

Indicators of Suicide Risk

- Lack of social support
- Social isolation
- Alienation from others
- Substance abuse
- Previous suicide attempts
- Inadequate coping skills
- Death or illness of significant others

Most research shows that lack of social support, social isolation or social alienation, substance abuse, previous suicide attempts, inadequate coping skills, and death or illness of significant others resulting from AIDS are all indicators of increased suicidal risk. One 1988 study by Marzuk and other researchers reported that gay men with AIDS in New York City were 36 times more likely to commit suicide than men without AIDS. By contrast, Brown and Rundell (1989) found that middle-class women who contracted HIV from heterosexual contact were at lower risk for suicide than men with HIV infection were at risk. While methods of completed suicide for persons with HIV infection vary, overdosing on drugs or medication may be the most common choice.

Philosophies and legality of "assisted" suicide are now being discussed in the context of a variety of terminal illnesses or seriously life-threatening disabilities, including HIV-related conditions. In fact, the 1996 XI International Conference on AIDS included several anecdotal reports and studies pointing to an increasing acceptance of assisted suicide. Given the current legal questions regarding assisted suicide, professionals in general tend not to directly participate in the act, and mental health professionals, in particular, are legally bound to prevent suicide (Wood, Marks, and Dilley, 1990). However, physicians may write prescriptions for a variety of narcotic medications which may facilitate their availability for overdose.

Risk Factors and Predictors Related to HIV/AIDS

Persons with HIV experience many sources of stress in their daily lives, most of which have also been identified as stressors by the general population. For example, Holmes and Rahe (l967) reported a listing of "life events" that were rated as stressful in a survey of a large number of people. These "events" were used to construct their "Social Readjustment Rating Scale." Ten of the top 17 events identified by the general population as stressful (e.g., death of a spouse, death of a close family member or friend, personal illness or injury, change in health, loss of job, or change in financial status) are commonly experienced by persons infected with HIV.

As the course of the illness progresses, HIV-infected persons frequently lose loved ones, they may be forced to give up jobs, their standard of living drops, they change residences, and they may experience declining health status that further debilitates both psychologically and physically. However, because there are multiple stages of HIV/AIDS disease, risk factors associated with suicidal thoughts or behavior often play differing roles during different stages.

Stages of HIV Disease

The following list and discussion elaborates three phases of HIV disease from a psychological perspective (Goldblum and Moulton, 1990).

Psychological Stages of HIV Disease

1. Initial Phase:

   –Dread, shock, and anger over news of infection

2. Middle Phase:

   –Beginning symptoms of AIDS

   –Breakdown of defenses, thoughts of death and suffering emerge

3. Final Phase:

   –Physical and mental deterioration with disability, disfigurement, and increased dependence on others

   (Goldblum and Moulton, 1990)

1. Initial Phase: According to Goldblum and Moulton (1990), one-half of the persons who receive the news of their HIV-positive status experience an acute crisis state with feelings of dread, shock, and anger. At the point of initial diagnosis, the person may use a range of defenses varying from denial, intrusive thoughts and psychic numbing, to feeling overwhelmed and confused. The person may be uncertain about the meaning of the test result and implications for future health status. Suicide risk may be increased if the person lacks information about the nature of the disease, is unaware of available resources, and lacks a strong emotional support system and financial resources.

2. Middle Phase: During the middle phase, the person may progress from being asymptomatic to experiencing initial symptoms. Defenses may break down, and thoughts of death and suffering may emerge. At this time, the person becomes more uncertain about the future. As the disease progresses and the person experiences new symptoms, he or she is faced with the impending diagnosis of AIDS, and psychological distress increases. Tross and Hirsch (1988) point out that, as people become more susceptible to opportunistic infection, suicidal thoughts are common, but death by suicide is rare. When a client is admitted to a critical care setting during an acute stage of illness, a crisis may develop and lead to feelings of intense helplessness, denial, anxiety, anger, and increased suicide risk.

3. Final Phase: Physical and mental deterioration progress with new and repeated infections that respond poorly to treatment. With the diagnosis of AIDS, thoughts of suicide may increase. If the person experiences symptoms of AIDS-related dementia, symptoms of depression and anger may be exacerbated. During the advanced stage of the illness, the person faces disability and disfigurement, increasing dependence on others, and difficulty in coping with daily liv-

ing. As the person is confronted with issues of pain, suffering, dependency, and loss of bodily functions, he or she realizes that death is imminent. The person may now see suicide as relief from suffering and a way of relieving others of the burden of care.

As the HIV-infected person enters the final or terminal stage, he or she may manifest some of the characteristics common to terminally ill persons who successfully commit suicide. Farberow, Schneidman, and Leonard (1970) have identified several of these characteristics including: exhaustion of physical and emotional resources; emotional stress increased by physiological stress; significantly more complaints of discomfort and pain; near-death physical condition; increased drug and alcohol abuse; and a history of suicide attempts.

Crisis Intervention and Suicide Risk Assessment

In addition to identifying HIV-related risk factors, mental health providers need to apply the basic principles of crisis intervention to guide the assessment and treatment of persons with HIV-related suicide intentions. Crisis intervention should include: listening to and understanding a person's story, assessing suicide risk, developing a crisis management plan, and closing with appropriate referrals for treatment. The clinical assessment includes an evaluation of the severity of the crisis, current suicide plan, coping patterns and strengths, social and personal resources, previous attempts, the lethality of the present plan or attempt, mental and medical status, and life-style.

Identifying Stressors and Exploring a Client's Intent

In assessing the severity of a crisis, it is important to identify specific stressors that have occurred within the past three weeks or so, especially those related to HIV. Additional stressors caused by HIV and AIDS are similar to those identified for persons with other chronic or life-threatening illnesses who may also exhibit an increased risk for suicide (Martin and Range, 1991).

Goldblum and Moulton (1990) identified these stressors as: multiple HIV-related losses; intimate involvement with another person who has died of AIDS; social ostracism (i.e., insults, discrimination, or injury related to fear of AIDS or homophobia); loss or restriction of employment; eviction or change of residence; loss of insurance coverage; painful and disfiguring physical deterioration; repeated infections; treatment failures; elaborate infection control procedures; exhaustion of financial resources; reliance on public assistance; and lack or loss of social support. These additional stressors should be examined on the basis of which of the three stages described earlier is occurring at the time the stressor occurs.

Other hazards can be situational events, such as a recent loss, anniversary date of the death of a significant other, a job change, rejection related to HIV or sexual orientation, or other events identified as meaningful by the client. It is essential to identify the event, discover the meaning of the event to the client, and obtain a clear description of the event.

There are also risk factors specific to gay men that occur when they are diagnosed as HIV-positive and their life-style is publicly exposed.

Suicide Risk Factors for HIV-Infected Gay Men

- Personal histories related to homophobia

    –Family history of rejection, history of employment or legal problems related to being gay

- A prevailing attitude that "the world is a dangerous place to be gay"

- Remaining *in the closet*

    –Engaging in homosexual behavior but avoiding identification with the gay community

- An unsettled sexual identity

    –Uncertainty in adolescents who feel that they may be gay

The above list is drawn from a discussion of specific risk factors for gay people with HIV, described by Goldblum and Moulton (1990) and based on clinical experience working with HIV-infected gay men.

Hoff (1984) made the useful point that signs or clues to suicide appear in different degrees among those who attempt suicide, those who succeed, and the general population. For example, recent loss happens to everyone and is generally resolved. However, it is an event that increases the risk of completed suicide for someone who has attempted suicide previously. Understanding the potential increase in suicide risk brought about by various social and psychological factors can aid the clinician in determining the risk of suicide.

The assessment of the crisis state includes exploring the client's symptoms and feelings, specifically, the severity of the symptoms. At this point, the counselor elicits information about the client's suicidal feelings, thoughts, and symptoms of depression to determine the degree of destabilization and manifestation of acute crisis symptoms. The more overwhelmed, helpless, and hopeless a person feels, the greater the risks.

The following questions may be asked in an assessment interview.

Questions to Ask the Client

- Have you thought of suicide?
- What did you think you might do?
- Do you have the means?
- Have you ever attempted suicide?
- Has anyone in your family attempted suicide?
- You said that you would be better off dead. Why do you feel this way?
- How do you see yourself in the future?
- What plans, if any, have you made concerning this action?
- Have you ever had ideas like this at any other time?
- Do you feel that these feelings could go away if you were given help?
- What help would you choose if it were available?
- What did you wish would happen when you attempted suicide?
- How do you feel now?
- What do you wish would happen now?

Look for verbal and behavioral warnings as listed below.

Verbal and Behavioral Predictors of Suicidal Behavior

- Verbal warnings
    - –Overt: "I'm going to kill myself."
    - –Covert: "I wish I were dead."
        "The only way out for me is to die."
        "Life has lost its meaning for me."
        "It's just too much to put up with."
        "Nobody needs me anymore."
        "I just can't go on any longer."
- Behavioral warnings
    - –Getting affairs in order

-Giving away cherished objects in a casual manner

-Previous suicide attempts

-Poor adjustment to the recent loss of a loved one

-Composing suicide notes

-Writing a will

-Asking about donating body to science

-Sudden, unexplainable recovery from a severe depression

-Purchasing or acquiring a gun or other lethal instrument

-Engaging in risk-taking behaviors, such as driving too fast

Verbal and behavioral warnings should always be treated seriously. Once the counselor suspects that someone is potentially suicidal, the best procedure is to approach the person in a warm, accepting, nonjudgmental manner and state something similar to "It sounds as if you are thinking about committing suicide" or "It sounds as if you may be thinking of killing yourself." Do not challenge the client or dare someone to commit suicide.

When asked if they intend to commit suicide, most suicidal people will answer honestly. Counselors should not avoid asking for fear of planting the idea in the mind of someone who never thought of it. If the person is feeling suicidal, discussing this with the counselor might provide such a strong catharsis that the situation is defused.

After the person has admitted to being at risk, the counselor assesses the degree of risk as soon as possible. To do that, the counselor asks the proper questions, in the right order. Is this an emergency? Does the counselor need to take steps immediately? The most efficient way is to determine if the person has a specific plan. An extremely poor question to begin with would be: "Why would you want to do something like that?" Instead, begin the assessment by asking "How?" (i.e., "How would you harm yourself?"). The answer to that question indicates the specificity of the plan. Without such a plan, the client is much less likely to take action immediately.

For persons acting on an impulse to kill themselves, their imagination is often clouded by mental anguish so their methods may involve whatever method is closest at hand. For example, prescription medications on the nightstand or in the medicine cabinet, a gun in the closet, or an open window or balcony may increase the possibility of impulsive suicide. A report on suicides in New York City in the mid-1980s indicated that about 5–7 percent of all AIDS-related deaths in one large clinical practice were suicides (Smith, 1989). The same article reported that one-quarter of the suicides of HIV or AIDS patients in the city were accomplished by jumping out of hospital windows, often shortly after receiving disheartening information about their medical status.

Persons who have taken great care to plan their death also use a variety of methods. For these individuals, detection of the suicide plan in time to intervene is often impossible. When the intervention is successful, it is because someone noticed the person engaged in behavior like "putting their affairs in order" or "becoming unusually calm and relaxed following a prolonged period of distress or grief." This calmness is the result of a reduction in stress that accompanies the decision to commit suicide.

Exploring the Seriousness of a Suicide Plan

It is important to assess the seriousness of a client's suicide risk. The counselor should ask the client whether he or she has ever thought of suicide and if there is a suicide plan. If the person does have a suicide plan, the counselor can use the acronym "ALPS," shown on the following list, to remember the first four factors that determine the seriousness of the risk. All four factors of the plan—availability, lethality, proximity, and specificity—should be assessed to determine the appropriate intervention.

Exploring the Seriousness of the Suicide Plan

> A = Availability
>
> L = Lethality
>
> P = Proximity
>
> S = Specificity

To explore the seriousness of the client's suicide plan, first inquire about the availability of the proposed method and whether the person has a realistic plan. If the proposed method is easily available, the risk is higher. Second, consider the lethality level of the proposed method. The more lethal the method, the higher the risk. Inquire as to how lethal the suicidal person believes the method would be; sometimes the suicidal person may not be aware that the method would not kill them. Third, determine the proximity of a potential rescuer. Has the suicidal person considered ways of preventing outside assistance or rescue? Has the person developed a plan where someone will be near to help prevent the suicide? The risk increases when helping resources are not close. Fourth, ask questions about the plan to determine the level of specificity. The more details that the person can identify, the higher the risk.

Assessing Coping Skills

Once the counselor assesses the client's immediate intent, his or her current and past coping strategies should be considered. This will help to determine how the individual will manage the present situation. Assess how the person coped before the HIV diagnosis, what his or her level of impulse control is, how he or she has tried to cope with the present situation and HIV-related stressors, what strategies have been successful, and what the person thinks would reduce feelings of stress or relieve the situation. Maladaptive coping mechanisms that increase suicide risk include alcohol and drug use, violent expression of anger and frustration, poor impulse control, and impaired judgment. Risk increases for persons who have limited or inadequate capacities to deal with stress. The counselor should explore whether the person uses HIV community resources and social supports.

Other researchers (Farberow, Schneidman, and Leonard, 1970) have pointed out that the most intolerable components of emotional distress tend to be rumination, negative thinking, and preoccupation with stressful situations. Typically, the time in which a person is most vulnerable to suicide lasts only a few seconds. Coping skills help people survive those seconds. These skills include those that are maladaptive, such as substance abuse or violence, and those that are adaptive, such as use of social supports, employment, caring for others, and recreational activities (Houston and Nuehring, 1988).

Significant others are those on whom the person relies for understanding and support when in distress. It is useful to identify the significant others and explore whether these relationships have deteriorated recently. Persons with HIV may feel rejected by their significant others because of the stigma attached to sexual orientation, injecting drug use, and HIV itself. The counselor must determine whether the client's perceptions are congruent with those of the significant others.

Social and personal resources facilitate an individual's functioning in the environment. These include adequate physical and mental capacities, having enough money, the proximity or availability of significant others, job, or hobbies, and necessities such as food, housing, clothing, healthcare facilities, and transportation. These resources can be depleted or unavailable for persons with HIV. The suicide risk is lowered by mobilizing these resources (Hatton and Valente, 1984; Maltsberger, 1986). As noted earlier, persons with HIV may encounter numerous losses such as death of HIV-infected partners, family, and friends; ostracism by others; job loss; and deterioration of health. When the precipitating event involves a significant object loss, the suicide risk increases. The lack of a social support network heightens feelings of worthlessness and self-depreciation. Emotional or physical isolation increases lethality.

In addition to assessing emotions, it is important to assess the activity level of the depressed person and to identify common symptoms of depression including insomnia, loss of sex drive, apathy, social withdrawal, helplessness, and hopelessness. A depressed person who feels helpless to change his or her situation and, at the same time, shows the restless expression of anxiety, guilt, or hostility is more likely to act on self-destructive impulses. As a severely depressed person's mood improves, his or her suicide potential may increase. The severely depressed may not have the energy to implement a suicide plan. As the depression lifts, the energy level increases. However, the feelings of hopelessness may remain and, coupled with increased activity, may result in an increased suicide risk. Also, a person who has made a commitment to a plan may feel relieved and appear less depressed.

If a person has a history of serious past pre-HIV or post-HIV suicide attempts, the lethality of his or her present suicidal crisis increases (Farberow, Schneidman, and Leonard, 1970; Hatton and Valente, 1984; Maltsberger, 1986). Find out if there have been any previous attempts, the means used, and how long ago the attempt occurred. The more recent the previous attempts, and the more lethal the means, the higher the current risk.

A person in crisis represents a more immediate suicide risk than a person with long-standing problems who is not in a crisis state. People with established histories of symptoms, such as substance abuse or depression, are more likely to survive the present episode, although they have a poorer long-term prognosis.

It is essential to collect information about a person's history of psychiatric problems both before and after HIV diagnosis. Potential clues to the current need for psychiatric treatment or hospitalization is often determined by whether or not those interventions were used successfully to alleviate symptoms or risk of suicide in the past. It is also important to assess past psychiatric intervention and counseling in view of how the client feels about past help. Note, however, that the absence of a psychiatric history does not necessarily indicate greater stability. The counselor should always ask questions about the person's current mental health and medical status. Acute or chronic physical illness often reduces the person's ability to cope. The counselor should look for symptoms of AIDS-related dementia and identify the impact of current physical symptoms.

A suicide risk assessment should include exploration of the client's feelings about his or her symptoms, disease progression, death and dying, and feelings of helplessness and hopelessness. Persons who have made end-of-life decisions beforehand will tend to feel more control over HIV disease. Information from collateral sources (such as physicians) is also helpful in determining prognosis and imminence of death. As noted earlier, each stage of the disease poses specific risks that should be assessed.

"Life-style" is defined as the maintenance and quality of the individual's interpersonal relationships, coping strategies, and job. The risk of suicide is reduced by a stable life-style. A person with a chronically unstable life-style is more vulnerable and may have difficulty coping with future stressful situations. It is important to evaluate the person's pre- and post-HIV life-style. As HIV treatment regimens become more holistic (e.g., emphasis on maintenance of a balanced life-style, the use of exercise, self-help and support groups, and stress management), persons who have already developed, or who can learn, healthy coping skills often pose a lower risk.

Immediate versus Long-Term Risks

Another step in assessment involves differentiating between an "immediate" and a "long-term" risk. An immediate risk is defined as the potential for the person to commit suicide within the next 24 hours. This is an emergency situation. Long-term risk is the likelihood a person may kill himself or herself within the next two years (Hatton and Valente, 1984).

The four-factor assessment of the seriousness of the suicide plan, ALPS (availability, lethality, proximity, specificity), can help determine the extent of the emergency. For example, a person may have a high or low ALPS score with reference to their suicide plan. However, presence of a stable life-style and available coping strategies for a person who feels suicidal with a highly lethal method available (a high ALPS score) would indicate an immediate risk. Persons who are long-term risks tend to have unstable life-styles, limited or destructive coping strategies, a history of suicide attempts, fleeting thoughts of suicide, but an unclear suicide plan (low ALPS score).

High ALPS = immediate risk

1. Available highly lethal method
2. Serious plan
3. Currently in crisis
4. Breakdown in coping strategies

Low ALPS = long-term risk

1. Fleeting thoughts of suicide
2. Unclear plan
3. Unstable lifestyle
4. Limited coping strategies
5. History of suicide attempts

Interventions are determined by these two kinds of ratings—immediate or long-term. A person at immediate risk may need hospitalization and may be amenable to crisis intervention, whereas long-term risk requires ongoing treatment and more comprehensive services.

Suicide Intervention

The task of the counselor is to develop an intervention based on assessment of suicidal risk. Ultimately, this becomes a clinical task for which there is significant liability. For that reason, the evaluator must have appropriate credentials, training, and supervision. In addition, detailed documentation of each phase of the assessment and intervention is essential. Be aware of any specific requirements of your facility and state, and always consult with your supervisor to review your plan. If the life-threatening behavior has already occurred, the professional's first priority is to ensure that the person receives medical treatment. Also, steps must be taken by the police, counselor, client, or significant others to eliminate the availability of any lethal or harmful means.

Once the person is safe, the professional counselor can guide the client in exploring alternatives to suicide. Attention must be given to helping the client express his or her fears, feelings, and concerns about the precipitating event and HIV status.

Interventions need to emphasize referral, linkages, and problem-solving efforts. Clients may need a medical evaluation for psychotropic medication or for the treatment of HIV-related symptoms. Additional interventions, such as family interviews, a contract, involuntary and voluntary hospitalization, referral, and follow-up may be needed. In determining referral needs, consideration should be given to daily, concrete, social, and psychological factors. Referrals may be needed for food, housing, medical care, etc. Social isolation should be reduced by building a viable support network of friends, family, volunteers, and other support groups.

Persons with HIV who are depressed and suicidal tend to respond best to a concerned, accepting, supportive therapeutic relationship. Expression of "unacceptable" thoughts is important; they need to understand and work through ambivalent feelings about death that they customarily have; they may need to grieve over losses. Family therapy may be an appropriate adjunct, and efforts to reduce social isolation through involvement with social groups and significant others are recommended. However, the critical treatment will probably occur in a supportive, longer term clinical relationship.

Some people believe that suicide is an acceptable choice that individuals have the right to make for themselves. Organizations like the Hemlock Society have existed for more than ten years to support the idea that persons with terminal illness have the right to commit suicide as a form of voluntary euthanasia. However, most professional ethical codes of conduct require practitioners to "do no harm." If the counselor feels unable to intervene to prevent a suicide attempt by persons facing terminal illness, he or she may consider whether it is appropriate to work with this population. At a minimum, the counselor must seek consultation and supervision.

At present, attention is being placed upon death with dignity and a client's right to self-determination. Healthcare alternatives, such as hospice, allow terminally ill persons to die without measures to prolong life while providing pain management. The "Federal Patient's Self Determination Act" of 1990 mandated healthcare facilities to inform patients of the facility's and state's policies regarding end-of-life decisions and advanced directives with no life support. Given these changes and the increased awareness of assisted suicide, professional organizations such as the National Association of Social Workers are beginning to address the professional's role in end-of-life decisions. Professional codes of ethics and policies continue to prohibit the mental health professional from participating in a client's assisted suicide. However, the professional can help the client explore alternatives such as hospice, advanced directives, and living wills. HIV-positive clients should be helped in expressing their feelings and thoughts about their impending death. To date, the mental health professional's role has been to help the client make informed decisions without sanctioning suicide (Wood, Marks, and Dilley, 1990).

Review Questions

1. Explain how a diagnosis of a terminal illness may affect suicide risk.

2. What does research on suicide risk for persons with HIV or AIDS indicate?

3. Name an activity that is a likely behavioral warning that a person plans to commit suicide.

4. Explain what the acronym "ALPS" means and what a high ALPS score indicates.

References and Suggested Readings

Alfonso, C.A., Cohen, M.A., Aladjem, A.D., Morrison, F., Powell, D.R., Winters, R.A., & Orlowski, B.K. (1994). HIV seropositivity as a major risk factor for suicide in the general hospital. *Psychosomatics, 35*(4), 368–373.

Biller, R., & Rice, S. (1990). Experiencing multiple loss of persons with AIDS. *Social Work, 35,* 283–290.

Bindels, P.J.E., Krol, A., van Ameijden, E., Mulder-Folkerts, D.K.F., van den Hoek, J.A.R., van Griensven, G.P.J., & Coutinho, R.A. (1996). Euthanasia and physician-assisted suicide in homosexual men with AIDS. *Lancet, 347,* 499–504.

Brown, G., & Rundell, J. (1989). Suicidal tendencies in women with human immunodeficiency virus infection. *American Journal of Psychiatry, 146*(4), 556–557.

Brown, G., & Rundell, J. (1990). Prospective study of psychiatric morbidity in HIV-seropositive women without AIDS. *General Hospital Psychiatry, 12*(1), 30–35.

Cote, R., Biggar, R., & Dannenberg, A. (1992). Risk of suicide among persons with AIDS: A national assessment. *Journal of the American Medical Association, 268,* 2066–2068.

Coleman, E., & Remafedi, G. (1989). Gay, lesbian, and bisexual adolescents: A critical challenge to counselors. Special Issue: Gay, lesbian, and bisexual issues in counseling. *Journal of Counseling and Development, 68*(1), 36–40.

Farberow, N.L., Helig, S.M., & Parad, H.J. (1990). Suicide prevention center: Concepts and clinical functions. In H.J. Parad, & L.G. Parad (Eds.), *Crisis Intervention Book 2: The Practitioner's Sourcebook for Brief Therapy.* (251–274). Milwaukee, WI: Family Service of America.

Farberow, N.L., Schneidman, E.S., & Leonard, C.V. (1970). Suicide among patients with malignant neoplasms. In E. Schneidman, N. Farberow, & P. Litman (Eds.), *Psychology of Suicide.* (325–344). New York: Science House.

Frierson, R., & Lippman, S. (1988). Suicide and AIDS. *Psychosomatics, 29*(2), 226–231.

Goldblum, P., & Moulton, J. 1989. HIV disease and suicide. In J.W. Dilley, C. Pies, & M. Helquist (Eds.), *Face to Face: A Guide to AIDS Counseling.* San Francisco: AIDS Health Project, University of California.

Hall, J.M., & Stevens, P.E. (1988). AIDS: A guide to suicide assessment. *Archives of Psychiatric Nursing, 2,* 115–120.

Hatton, C., & Valente, S. (Eds.) (1984). *Suicide: Assessment and Intervention* (2nd ed.). East Norwalk, CT: Appleton-Century-Crofts.

Hoff, L. (1984). *People in Crisis: Understanding and Helping.* Menlo Park, CA: Addison-Wesley.

Holmes, T.H., & Rahe, R.N. (1967). The Social Readjustment Rating Scale. *Journal of Psychosomatic Research, ll,* 213–218.

Houston, M., & Nuehring, E. (1988). *Screener's Handbook for Mental Health Emergency Intervention.* Unpublished manuscript, Barry University Research and Training Center. Miami Shores, FL.

Kaisch, K., & Anton-Culver, H. (1989). Psychological and social consequences of HIV exposure: Homosexual in Southern California. *Psychology and Health, 3*(2), 63–75.

Kizer, K., Green, M., Perkins, C., Doebbert, G., & Hughes, M. (1988). AIDS and suicide in California. *Journal of the American Medical Association, 260,* 1881–1882.

Kubler-Ross, E. (1977). *On Death and Dying.* New York: Macmillan.

Maltsberger, J.T. (1986). *Suicide Risk: The Formulation of Clinical Judgment.* New York: New York University Press.

Mancoske, R.J., Wadsworth, C.M., Dugas, D.S., & Hasney, J.A. (1995). Suicide risk among people living with AIDS. *Social Work, 40,* 783–787.

Martin, S., & Range, L. (1991). Extenuating circumstances in perceptions of suicide: Disease diagnosis (AIDS, cancer), pain level, and life expectancy. *Omega, 22,* 187–197.

Marzuk, P., Tierney, H., Tardiff, K., Gross, E., Morgan, E., Hsu, M., & Mann, J. (1988). Increased risk of suicide in persons with AIDS. *Journal of the American Medical Association, 260,* 1333–1337.

McKegney, F., & O'Dowd, M. (1992). Suicidality and HIV status. *American Journal of Psychiatry, 149*(3), 396–398.

Neugebauer, R., & Johnson, J. (1990). Does HIV testing raise levels of suicidal ideation? *Journal of the American Medical Association, 264*(3), 337–338.

O'Dowd, M., & McKegney F. (1990). AIDS patients compared with others seen in psychiatric consultation. *General Hospital Psychiatry, 12*(1), 50–55.

O'Dowd, M.A., Biderman, D.J., & McKegney, F.P. (1993). Incidence of suicidality in AIDS and HIV-positive patients attending a psychiatry outpatient program. *Psychosomatics, 34*(1), 33–40.

Plott, R., Benton, S., & Winslade, W. (1989). Suicide of AIDS patients in Texas: A preliminary report. *Texas Medicine, 85*(8), 40–43.

Ryan, C. (1988). The social and clinical challenges of AIDS. Special Issue: AIDS. *Smith College Studies in Social Work, 59*(1), 3–20.

Saunders, J., & Buckingham, S. (1988). Suicidal AIDS patients: When the depression turns deadly. *Nursing, 18*(7), 59–64.

Schneidman, E., Farberow, N., & Litman, P. (Eds.) (1970). *Psychology of Suicide.* New York: Science House.

Schneider, S., Taylor, S., Hammen, C., Kemeny, M., & Dudley, J. (1991). Factors influencing suicide intent in gay and bisexual suicide ideators: Different models for men with and without human immunodeficiency virus. *Journal of Personality and Social Psychology, 61*(5), 776–788.

Smith, K. (l989). AIDS suicide: Ultimate choice or desperate act? *Patient Care,* August, 20–22.

Tross, S., & Hirsch, D. (1988). Psychological distress and neuropsychological complications of HIV infection and AIDS. *American Psychologist, 43*(11), 929–934.

van Haastrecht, H.J., Mientjes, G.H., van den Hoek, A.J., & Coutinho, R.A. (1994). Death from suicide and overdose among drug injectors after disclosure of first HIV test result. *AIDS, 8*(12), 1721–1725.

Waldinger, R.J. (1986). *Fundamentals of Psychiatry.* Washington, D.C.: American Psychiatric Press.

Westermeyer, J., Seppala, M., Gasow, S., & Carlson, G. (1989). AIDS-related illness and AIDS risk in male homo/bisexual substance abusers: Case reports and clinical issues. *American Journal of Drug and Alcohol Abuse, 15*(4), 443–461.

Wood, G., Marks, R., & Dilley, J. (1990). *AIDS Law for Mental Health Professionals.* Berkeley, CA: Celestial Arts Press.

Chapter 14

Preparing for Death

Jeremy S. Gaies, Psy.D., and
Michael D. Knox, Ph.D.

Overview

This chapter on preparing for death provides an introduction to issues relevant to clients who have HIV disease. Assessment guidelines and therapeutic interventions for clients and families who are coping with a diagnosis of terminal illness are reviewed. Suggestions for preventing provider burnout are included. The focus of community mental health treatment is delineated.

Learning Objectives

1. To identify essential elements in the mental health assessment of clients with terminal HIV disease.

2. To describe therapeutic goals and interventions for mental health treatment of persons with terminal HIV disease.

3. To list factors affecting partners, families, and others who are facing the loss of a loved one with HIV disease.

4. To specify techniques for avoiding and reducing provider burnout.

5. To explain the role of hospice care and other community resources in the care of persons with terminal HIV disease.

Outline

Terminal Aspects of HIV Disease

HIV disease is increasingly being treated and viewed as a condition that can be managed over time. At present, however, AIDS remains life-threatening. Understanding the issues of death and dying that are raised by HIV disease is therefore important for community mental health center (CMHC) staff.

Preparing the Client

During the past eighteen years in the United States alone, AIDS has claimed the lives of nearly 400,000 people. More than 60 percent of the individuals diagnosed with the disease have died. Statistics suggest that most people currently diagnosed with AIDS will die as a result of the condition. Issues regarding death and dying are raised not only for those persons with AIDS, but for the many persons infected with HIV who are not yet showing any symptoms. There continues to be no reliable means for predicting longevity for individuals with HIV disease. Many people, even those with CD4 cell counts below 200, live for years. The goal of preparing clients is to help them accept the possibility, not the inevitability, of a premature death.

Assessment

The first, and perhaps most important, step in providing care is to conduct a thorough assessment. Assessment of persons with AIDS is challenging because there are many special areas to assess and because issues of the illness—including its modes of transmission and its terminal nature—can raise strong emotional responses in health and mental healthcare providers.

Assessment Guidelines

■ *Select* a framework.
  –Be sure the framework is *objective.*
  –Be sure the framework is *comprehensive.*
  –Be sure the framework is *broad-based.*

■ *Practice* applying the framework.
  –Assessment should *respect the client's privacy.*
  –Assessment should include *terminal issues.*
  –Assessment should be *ongoing.*

It is important to select a framework for assessment that is objective, comprehensive, and broad-based. Objectivity is important, given the emotional nature of the subject, including issues of mortality. Comprehensiveness allows a full review of often avoided areas. A broad-based approach to assessment assures attention to the various levels at which a client may be functioning: emotional, behavioral, and neuropsychological. A structured clinical interview that includes a specific focus on terminal issues can serve as an appropriate framework.

Providers can benefit by practicing the use of such a framework in training and with clients to gain familiarity and comfort with the format. The more comfortable the provider is with the structure, the more comfortable the client is likely to be in providing the requested information. Assessment should always respect the client's right to privacy as well as confidentiality. Clients should not be pressured to discuss issues that they do not feel comfortable discussing at that time. Assessment should, however, include specific focus on terminal issues, allowing clients who do wish to discuss fears or issues regarding the dying process a direct invitation to speak about these feelings. Lastly, assessment should be ongoing. Issues, and readiness to discuss them, change with time. Several opportunities should be given to collect the information that can assist treatment.

Key Areas of Assessment

There are many areas that are essential to a thorough assessment of the client with advanced AIDS. A brief look at the following diagram helps to illustrate the many areas that may have an impact upon the person with advanced HIV disease.

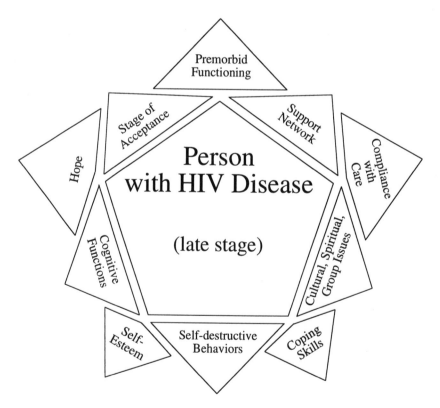

FIGURE 14.1 Key areas of assessment.

All of these components should be part of the initial or ongoing assessment.

Premorbid functioning refers to the client's level of functioning before he or she was identified as HIV-positive, before he or she was diagnosed with AIDS, or before the current psychological symptoms began. Assessing the premorbid functioning allows a comparison with current functioning to identify the degree of change.

A support network includes partners, family, friends, professionals, and others with whom the client has a bond. A strong support network can serve many functions, including monitoring care, providing emotional and practical support, and preventing isolation.

Compliance with care includes compliance with medication regimens, both those for AIDS and those for other medical and psychiatric conditions. It also includes maintaining self-care through adequate hygiene, nutrition, and sleep.

Cultural, spiritual, and group issues include any issues related to a client's culture, subculture, religion, spiritual beliefs, or group identifications. Racial, ethnic, and religious factors can be highly influential to a person's coping style, as can be factors specific to gender or sexual orientation. Ethnic and religious influences on coping with the dying process from both the patient's and the bereaved's perspectives should be particularly noted.

Coping skills should be examined to determine both the degree to which a person possesses them and the degree to which they are using them. Obstacles to the use of current coping skills can be explored. Skills that are normally adequate may be inadequate when confronted with issues of terminal disease.

The risk of self-destructive behaviors, especially suicide, must be assessed. Suicide risk, based on past suicide attempts, current ideation and plan, psychological factors (such as impulsivity and current level of hopelessness), and related risk factors (such as substance abuse and isolation) should be evaluated. (See Chapter 13, "Suicide Assessment and Intervention with Persons Infected with HIV.") Other self-destructive behavior should also be identified, including unsafe sexual practices.

Self-esteem, both premorbid and current, should be assessed. Low self-esteem may contribute to poor compliance with care, increased self-destructiveness, and inadequate use of coping skills. Terminal conditions may threaten self-esteem but can also present opportunities for enhancing self-esteem.

Changes in cognitive functions resulting from HIV must be evaluated thoroughly, especially with decreasing immune functioning and related illness. Neuropsychological status should be monitored. (See Chapter 9, "Neuropsychological Functioning in HIV Disease.")

Hope, optimism, and other positive buffers to stress and distress should be measured. Absence of these factors may contribute to suicide risk, self-destructiveness, noncompliance with treatment, and lack of resilience to depression. Bolstering these psychological buffers can have profound impact not only on coping but also on maintaining health status.

Lastly, it is useful to examine the client's current stage of acceptance of his or her condition and prognosis. A helpful guide for exploring these stages is the classic model proposed by Kubler-Ross (1969). Kubler-Ross proposed five stages—denial, anger, bargaining, depression, and acceptance—as an orderly progression starting from the original diagnosis of a terminal illness. While more recent research finds that these stages may not be so orderly or fixed, the model does suggest several emotional phases that clients may experience in a generally progressive manner.

Diagnostic Issues

The issues associated with dying may lead to symptoms of major depression, adjustment disorder, anxiety disorders, or other psychological dysfunction. Decompensation from stable functioning for persons with pre-existing mental disorders such as schizophrenia, bipolar disorder, recurrent major depression, or panic disorders, may also occur. (See Chapter 17, "Treating Persons with Serious and Persistent Mental Illness.")

Providers must be careful not to assume that the client's response is simply an exacerbation of a pre-existing disorder and, therefore, does not need a response specific to the symptoms. For example, a major depression superimposed on a pre-existing schizophrenic disorder will require similarly intense (if not greater) attention than a major depression in the absence of a pre-existing disorder. (See Chapter 12, "Depression and HIV Disease.") On the other hand, it is important to recognize that, at times, the stress of being diagnosed with a life-threatening illness may increase symptoms of pre-existing conditions. Treatment should then focus on restabilizing the client. For example, a client with a thought disorder may need an increase in his or her regular medication to maintain stable functioning in the midst of increased emotional stressors.

Intervention

Therapeutic Goals and Intervention Tasks

The primary goals of intervention include maintaining stable functioning, fostering the process of acceptance of the terminal condition and prognosis, and enhancing coping skills and social supports for upcoming challenges. These goals can be met by attending to the intervention tasks outlined here.

Therapeutic Goals

■ Maintain stable functioning.

- Foster client's acceptance of his or her diagnosis.
- Enhance coping skills.
- Increase social supports.

Intervention Tasks

- Foster communication.
- Enlist support.
- Foster individual empowerment.
- Assist in planning.
- Assure medical care.
- Assure psychological care.
- Teach coping skills.

The major intervention tasks in helping a client prepare for death include fostering communication, enlisting support from others, fostering individual empowerment, assisting in planning, assuring that medical and psychological needs are met, and teaching coping skills.

Fostering communication of information and feelings often includes skills training, behavioral rehearsal, or supportive encouragement. Encouragement may be needed for clients to ask questions about their medical care or to express feelings about their experience with the illness.

Helping clients enlist support from family and others includes facilitating communication of feelings and needs to partners, family, and friends and arranging for care assistance as physical or psychological health declines. It is important to recognize that social support systems vary. For example, for many gay men, partners and close friends form a stronger network than blood relatives. For many African Americans and Hispanics, extended family networks are heavily involved in an individual's life. Enlisting support also means gaining knowledge of relevant community resources.

Fostering individual empowerment is important because clients with AIDS lose so much control as a result of the disease. Offering clients the opportunity to make decisions is a way of fostering empowerment, even if the decisions are minor.

Planning tasks are many and may include a last will and testament; a living will; a durable power of attorney to assist the client when he or she is no longer able to make decisions, especially healthcare decisions; home healthcare options; hospice involvement; and provisions for dependent children. Clients may also wish to plan for their own funeral and memorial service and provide final instructions to their survivors. Making decisions, taking charge of the final details, and being creative in the process can enhance personal autonomy and self-esteem at a time when everything else seems out of control.

Assuring that medical, psychological, and other service needs are met begins during assessment, but may later require ongoing case management to assure continued provision of these services. Teaching coping skills, including relaxation, assertiveness, and pain management, can assist clients in managing stressful conditions related to their diagnosis and treatment.

Intervention Guidelines

Applying the intervention tasks may best be accomplished by following certain basic guidelines, as shown below:

Intervention Guidelines

- Be aware of client's cognitive status.
- Foster a safe emotional environment.
- Be clear and comfortable when discussing death and dying.
- Attend to key areas of assessment and intervention.
- Take time to listen.

Being aware of the client's cognitive status, i.e., the ability to comprehend, is essential. Two major potential obstacles to a client's ability to understand information fully are a pre-existing intellectual limitation and a current neuropsychological impairment resulting from HIV disease.

It is important not to push a client to feel one way or another, or to be at one stage or another. It is far more effective to foster a safe emotional environment that allows the client to progress naturally through the process toward acceptance. While we try to assist clients with acceptance of terminal illness, denial serves a useful purpose to help clients modulate the amount of information they can handle at any given time.

Do not be afraid to talk directly about death and dying. Use the words and allow the client's responses to be an indicator of how ready he or she is to discuss terminal issues. Your comfort and directness will often signal to the client that you are someone with whom it is safe to freely discuss feelings and fears.

Attend to the important areas of assessment and to the essential intervention tasks, as outlined previously. Finally, be prepared to take time to listen. Allowing the client to tell his or her story is an important part of the process of preparing for death.

Preparing the Bereaved: Partners, Family, Children, and Friends

The same issues that HIV-infected clients must address are, at times, also raised by partners, family members, and caregivers, including mental health caregivers.

Bereavement: Basic Issues

Bereavement is the natural process that we undergo when we lose something or someone important to us. Because the process is a natural and healthful one, it should not be prevented by stopping the expression of emotions or by ignoring the thoughts and feelings raised by the loss. The process cannot be speeded up, although it can be facilitated by creating an environment in which a bereaved person feels safe and is encouraged to express feelings and thoughts.

Bereavement: HIV-Specific Issues

People experiencing the process of bereavement for someone who has died or is dying of AIDS may have special issues to face. Stigma and secrecy regarding AIDS may prevent some people from openly expressing their sadness. Anger is commonly experienced, especially when a person feels that the disease or the death could have been prevented. Guilt is not uncommon when a bereaved person regrets their rejection of the HIV-infected person as a result of the person's sexual behavior, drug use, or mental illness.

Needs of the Bereaved

Partners, family members, and friends may experience aspects of the loss before the client's death if they are aware of the client's illness. The needs of the bereaved include preparing for the loss as well as coping with the loss when it occurs.

Needs of Bereaved That May Require Support

- Prior to client's death

    –Saying good-bye

    –Communicating feelings

     –Coping with the anticipated loss

     –Planning late-stage medical care (hospital, hospice, etc.)

     –Funeral and memorial planning

■ After the client's death

     –Grieving

     –Funeral and memorial planning (if not prearranged)

     –Attending to the client's estate and final instructions

     –Notifying individuals and agencies

     –Readjusting to life

Before the client's death, the needs of loved ones may focus on communicating with the client, coping with the anticipated loss, and making practical plans for final healthcare and a funeral, if the client is unable to do so independently. A special area of importance is saying good-bye, which individuals need to do in their own way. Some people say their good-byes verbally, nonverbally, or through their actions. Encouraging as direct communication as possible is often helpful. Supporting the bereaved as they say their good-byes is also frequently necessary.

After the client's death, the loved ones begin the process of grieving, but may initially need to attend to remaining practical details. These include planning for the funeral and memorial, if not prearranged; attending to the client's estate; and notifying appropriate individuals and agencies of the client's death. Readjusting to life is a long-term aspect of the bereavement process and may require months or years, depending upon a person's individual coping style and their relationship to the individual who died. Professional support is sometimes needed through this normal but sometimes difficult grief process.

In many cases, before the client's death, the needs of the client and the bereaved overlap. For example, helping the client to communicate with the family also helps meet the family's needs. In addition, any practical planning that can occur before the client's death assists the bereaved as well. *Last Wishes: A Handbook to Guide Your Survivors* (Knox and Knox, 1995), a workbook for recording funeral, memorial, and other final instructions, is a resource for such planning.

Preparing the Provider

Challenges of Terminal Care Treatment

As early as 1989, research data (Dow and Knox, 1989) began to suggest that staff discomfort in working with HIV-infected persons is comprised, in part, by discomfort with the issue of terminal illness. Treatment staff attributed their discomfort to their lack of training and the belief that little can be done to help a terminally ill person.

In fact, there is much that CMHC staff can do to help clients with terminal illnesses. Clinicians can provide assistance for clients who are living with the illness for as much time as he or she has to live. Working with dying clients can be difficult but can also be a very rewarding and inspiring professional experience.

Perhaps the most important guideline for a clinician working with dying patients is to work actively and consistently to prevent and resolve one's own emotional burnout.

Preventing and Resolving Care Provider Burnout

- Set reasonable expectations.
- Maintain a balance between work and play.
- Find support at work and home.
- Learn about HIV and the issues of death and dying.
- Consult with co-workers.
- Use humor.
- Practice stress management.
- Confront your own issues.
- Maintain personal and professional fulfillment.
- Say good-bye.

Burnout prevention is composed of many tasks. An important start is to set reasonable goals for treatment for the client. Part of this process involves learning to be patient with the sometimes slow pace of change. Maintaining diverse activities outside of your job, including physical exercise and activities that are fun, is important. Finding support among co-workers, family, and friends can give you an important emotional outlet. Learning more about HIV and how to handle death and dying can also prevent providers from feeling overwhelmed or not competent. Working with co-therapists, discussing feelings in case conferences or staff meetings, or talking informally with co-workers during breaks in the day can help act as a buffer.

Other burnout skills include using humor, practicing relaxation, exploring one's own feelings regarding death and the meaning of life, identifying achievable goals that add a sense of purpose to work, and focusing attention every day on personal fulfillment. Saying good-bye to clients, in some manner, is also important for those who work with dying persons.

Resources in Working with Persons with Late-Stage AIDS

Hospice Philosophy and Practice

The community mental health system has a very important role to play in meeting the needs of the terminally ill client with AIDS. As with medical care for a client who may die in a relatively brief period of time, the orientation of community mental health treatment may be less on producing long-term behavior changes and more on assisting a client to cope with the challenges of the remaining years, months, weeks, or days. This orientation fits well with the philosophy of the hospice movement. Hospice care focuses on enhancing client comfort and dignity rather than on curing a terminal or end-stage disease. Hospice services are broad, including home care, family respite, education, bereavement services, and, in some areas, an inpatient setting where patients may die in a comfortable, nonhospital setting that also provides nursing care.

Accessing Community Resources

Many community resources are available for persons with a terminal illness, their partners, and families. In addition to hospice organizations, AIDS service organizations, community support groups, and other community agencies, as well as some governmental and private nonprofit agencies, often provide low-cost or free services to assist persons with AIDS or other terminal conditions. Local AIDS service organizations should be able to refer families to funeral homes that are sympathetic to families who have lost someone to AIDS.

Review Questions

1. What are some important therapeutic interventions in preparing a client for death?

2. Describe some important skills that a bereavement counselor should possess.

3. How can a provider prevent burnout?

References and Suggested Readings

Anderson, P. (1991). *Affairs in Order: A Complete Resource Guide to Death and Dying.* New York: Macmillan.

Donnelley, K.F. (1994). *Recovering from the Loss of a Loved One to AIDS: Help for Surviving Family, Friends, and Lovers Who Grieve.* New York: St. Martin's Press.

Dow, M.G., & Knox, M.D. (1989). *Attitudes and Knowledge about AIDS and Administrative Impediments to Service in Florida's State-Funded Community Mental Health Centers and Drug Abuse Treatment Programs.* Tampa, FL: Florida Mental Health Institute.

Gaies, J., & Knox, M. (1991). The therapist and the dying client. *Focus: A Guide to AIDS Research and Counseling,* 6(6), 1–2.

Knox, L.P., & Knox, M.D. (1995). *Last Wishes: A Handbook to Guide Your Survivors.* Berkeley: Ulysses Press.

Kubler-Ross, E. (1993). *AIDS: The Ultimate Challenge.* New York: Macmillan.

Kubler-Ross, E. (1969). *On Death and Dying.* New York: Macmillan.

Martelli, L.J. (1993). *When Someone You Know Has AIDS.* New York: Crown Publishers.

Martin, J.P. (1991). Making terminal care decisions. *Focus: A Guide to AIDS Research and Counseling,* 6(6), 3.

Worden, J.W. (1991). *Grief Counseling and Grief Therapy: A Handbook for the Mental Health Practitioner* (2nd ed.). New York: Springer.

Part IV

Special Topics

Chapter 15

Women and HIV

Caroline H. Sparks, Ph.D.

Overview

This chapter provides information about the cultural and political factors that affect women who are at risk for HIV disease or those who already have the disease. It includes a discussion of special problems that community mental health center (CMHC) staff must consider when designing prevention or mental health programs for HIV-infected women. These problems include gender and racial discrimination, poverty, discrimination in the healthcare system, and social attitudes and practices that contribute to women's risk. Suggestions for prevention programs and mental health services are included.

Learning Objectives

1. To cite at least three cultural and political factors affecting women at risk for HIV disease.

2. To identify problems of HIV disease that are unique to women.

3. To demonstrate an understanding of issues that affect women's adoption of preventive behaviors.

4. To formulate a basic plan for helping women who are HIV-infected to access care in the local community.

Outline

I. Cultural and Political Factors Affecting Women at Risk for HIV Disease
   A. The epidemiology of AIDS among women
   B. The social context of HIV/AIDS

II. Disease Manifestations in Women, Treatment, and Decisions about Pregnancy
   A. Common manifestations in women
   B. Need for comprehensive treatment and follow-up
   C. Decisions about becoming pregnant

III. Promoting Preventive Behaviors for Women at Risk for HIV
   A. Psychological and social factors
      1. Fear of violence
      2. Importance of relationships with others
      3. Economic dependence
      4. Self-esteem
      5. Lack of social support
   B. Strategies for prevention for women
      1. Promoting good self-care
      2. Woman-focused preventive education
      3. Aggressive outreach to women who use drugs

IV. Helping Women with HIV Disease to Access Appropriate Medical and Mental Healthcare
   A. Assessing family and social support for women and their infected or uninfected children
   B. Locating and negotiating family-centered care
   C. Finding drug addiction treatment programs
   D. Providing support groups
V. Conclusion

Cultural and Political Factors Affecting Women at Risk for HIV Disease

Our ability to address the psychosocial and health problems confronting women with HIV disease requires an awareness of the social context within which women who are at risk, or who have the disease, live and make decisions. Sensitivity to the complex forms of inequality that women in our culture experience is important to a CMHC's development of appropriate programs for this population. Sexual, racial, and economic disparities in our society predate but are reflected in our response to women who have HIV disease. Understanding the social context in which HIV occurs among women requires a sensitivity on the part of CMHC staff to the impact of gender roles, drug subcultures, race, and class on women's lives.

The Epidemiology of AIDS among Women

By December 1996, women represented 20 percent of new AIDS cases and 15 percent of the cumulative total of cases in the United States, more than double the percentage of cases in 1987. Women of color represent 75 percent of AIDS cases in women. African-American women represent 55 percent and Hispanic women represent 20 percent of these cases, percentages far in excess of the representation of these groups in the general population. AIDS is the leading cause of death in young black women. Rates of HIV infection are highest for women who live in urban areas.

The two most important risk factors for women are using drugs or having sex with someone who uses drugs. As the following chart shows, the two major exposure routes for HIV in women have been injecting drug use (45%) and heterosexual contact (38%). Of those who have contracted the disease from heterosexual contact, 46 percent contracted HIV disease by having sex with an injecting drug user.

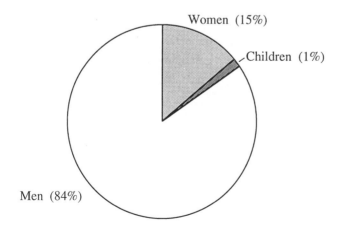

FIGURE 15.1 Cumulative AIDS cases, through December 1996, United States.

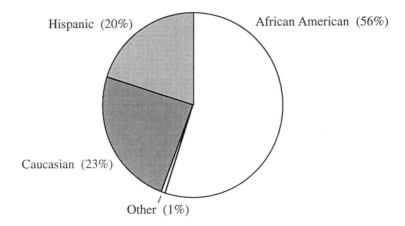

FIGURE 15.2 Cumulative AIDS cases in women by race/ethnicity, through December 1996, United States.

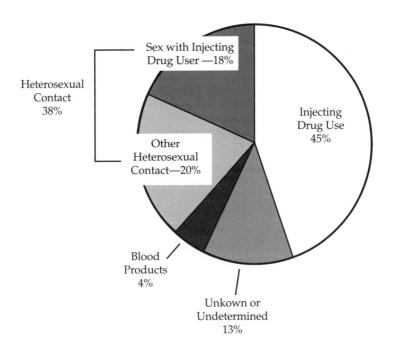

FIGURE 15.3 Cumulative AIDS cases in women by mode of transmission, through December 1996, United States.

Since HIV infection is the third leading cause of death for women between the ages of 25 and 44 years, the prevention and treatment of HIV disease and the emotional stresses that accompany it are a major health problem for women that will demand more attention as the epidemic continues. Limiting the risk of contracting HIV disease for women requires an understanding of the determinants of drug use among women as well as an understanding of the social context that influences women's decisions about relationships.

The Social Context of HIV/AIDS

Effective responses to HIV disease in women are impeded by several social problems that have a heavy impact on women who are most at risk for HIV.

Social Problems Affecting the Response to Women at Risk for HIV Disease

- Racial discrimination
- Sexual discrimination
- Poverty
- Punitive attitudes about women's sexual behavior and drug use
- Invisibility of lesbians and bisexual women as risk groups
- Discrimination in the healthcare system

Racial and sexual discrimination affect society's response to women's needs and, particularly, limit available resources for minority women. Since African-American and Hispanic women already suffer both racial and sexual discrimination, they bear this same double burden of discrimination when they contract HIV and attempt to secure medical, mental health, and social services.

The burden of HIV for these groups of women is made heavier by poverty. Economically, the women most at risk of HIV have the fewest resources to protect themselves from the disease or to obtain good healthcare. The majority of women who have contracted HIV through their own or their partners' drug use come from urban multiproblem families of lower socioeconomic status. Many have not completed high school. They may be working at low-paying positions with little security or be dependent upon male partners. Many women most at risk live by selling or trading sex for drugs. The women most affected by the disease are often isolated from community advocacy organizations and are not accustomed to participating in the political process in a way that would secure more resources for themselves.

They are often too overwhelmed by the demands of children, families, or their own dysfunction to begin their own community organizations. As a result, women with HIV have not developed an effective consumer lobby to direct public attention to their needs as have other groups, such as gay men.

Public disdain for women who use drugs or work in the sex trade has meant that women are likely to be held responsible for their own illness as well as for transmitting the disease to men or to their own children. Early in the AIDS epidemic, women who work in the sex trade were often cited as a major source of infection for men. In reality, women who trade or sell sex for drugs are at risk for HIV infection from customers and pimps who bribe, physically coerce, or use drugs as incentives to get women to engage in unprotected sex.

Another group of women at risk for HIV who experience prejudice and whose needs have received little attention are lesbian and bisexual women. For some years, the CDC listed cases of HIV in lesbians or bisexual women under the "unknown" or "undetermined" categories in surveillance reports. Although little is known about the national seroprevalence rates for lesbians and bisexual women, one recent study of 27,370 women seen in four New York State counseling and testing programs found an HIV seroprevalence of 3 percent in women sexually active exclusively with women and 4.8 percent in women sexually active with both women and men, compared with 2 percent for women sexually active exclusively with men. In this study, injecting drug use was the predominant risk factor for women (Shotsky, 1996). Special programs are needed to serve this population because services at women's health centers are often aimed at heterosexual women while services at gay health centers are often aimed at gay men.

All of the forms of prejudice mentioned—racial, gender, economic, and sexual orientation—constitute structural barriers that hinder the development of sensitive, appropriate services for women and that reduce women's access to care. Professionals working to stem the AIDS crisis have pointed out that our healthcare system reflects traditional sex discrimination against women as seen in exclusion from medical research, less adequate health insurance, and fewer targeted prevention and treatment programs.

Many women have difficulty securing medical treatment for AIDS because they have no health insurance. Business practices of hiring part-time employees to avoid paying employee benefits or paying illegal aliens "off the books" deprive many women of benefits. Women in entry level or clerical positions, or those who have low seniority, change jobs frequently and are excluded from insurance for varied periods by restrictions on pre-existing conditions. Even women who would otherwise qualify for insurance, once diagnosed with HIV disease, often become uninsurable.

Women still have problems accessing HIV care because the CDC's AIDS case definition continues to omit common symptoms found in women. Receiving an AIDS diagnosis broadens a woman's treatment options and helps her to establish eligibility for disability benefits. While the CDC's 1992 revision of the AIDS case definition helped some women with AIDS to be identified earlier, the new definition still did not recognize such common gynecological manifestations of AIDS in women as recurring pelvic inflammatory disease, recurrent yeast infections, and cervical cancers that have not yet become invasive. International definitions of AIDS also do not include medical conditions common to women, even though heterosexual transmission of HIV is the most common route of infection for women around the world.

Disease Manifestations in Women, Treatment, and Decisions about Pregnancy

Common Manifestations in Women

The following list shows some of the most common symptoms in women who are HIV-positive. Weight loss, anemia, and aching muscles and joints are frequent complaints, as is oral thrush.

Common Symptoms for Women Who Are HIV-Positive

- Weight loss
- Anemia
- Aching muscles and joints
- Oral thrush
- Recurring and persistent vaginal yeast infections
- Cervical dysplasia
- Cervical cancer
- Genital warts

The gynecological problems experienced by women have received more attention in the past several years as physicians recognized that the course of HIV disease in women differs from that in men. The five most common AIDS-defining illnesses in women are *Pneumocystis carinii* pneumonia, esophageal candidiasis, chronic ulcerative herpes, wasting, and *Mycobacterium avium-intracellulare* complex.

The 1992 CDC definition of AIDS recognized invasive cervical cancer as an AIDS-defining illness. Other common gynecological conditions create medical problems for women with HIV disease. They may experience recurrent vaginal yeast infections, which are often resistant to treatment. Cervical dysplasia, caused by the human papillomavirus (HPV), is often a preliminary condition to the development of cervical cancer. More research is needed on the relationship between HIV infection and cervical cancer. Women with HIV disease are often infected, as are men, with genital warts. However, in women, the recurrences are more frequent and pervasive and are more resistant to treatment than that in men.

Need for Comprehensive Treatment and Follow-up

Medical Needs of Women with HIV Disease

- HIV training for gynecologists
- Prevention information in ob/gyn offices
- PAP smears every six months and annual colposcopies
- Routine screening and treatment for sexually transmitted diseases (STDs)
- Treatment for common vaginal infections
- Comprehensive medical assessments
- Early medical intervention
- Education about risks to the immune system during pregnancy
- Regular follow-up care

This list identifies medical needs of women with HIV disease. One of the most important issues is access to appropriate medical care. Since the only physician that many women will see during the year is a gynecologist, these physicians must become primary sources for HIV preventive education and for early HIV screening for women.

STDs, which cause genital ulcers, such as syphilis, gonorrhea, chancroid, and herpes, are thought to increase the chance of HIV transmission between sexual partners. STDs need to be identified and treated to reduce the chances of HIV infection. Chlamydia and trichomoniasis, other common infections women contract during sexual relations with infected partners, may also increase vulnerability to HIV infection.

For women who are HIV-positive, PAP smears every six months and an annual colposcopy are indicated health measures. Cervical dysplasia can be treated early with cryosurgery, cauterization, or laser treatment.

Women with HIV disease need comprehensive medical assessments with regular follow-up care, which many, unfortunately, cannot afford and do not receive. Often women cannot or do not keep their appointments. The advent of new antiviral therapies, such as protease inhibitors, makes the need for regular medical checkups even more important. A CMHC may be able to help clients keep appointments by providing case management and arranging transportation. CMHCs may work with community health clinics to create accessible services for more women.

Decisions about Becoming Pregnant

Women with HIV disease must carefully weigh the consequences to their own health of becoming pregnant and carrying a child to term. During pregnancy, and for three months following delivery, a woman's immune system may be more vulnerable to HIV disease progression since her system must adapt to accept the fetus.

Sensitive counseling can raise a woman's awareness about the probability that a child born to a mother who is HIV-positive may be HIV-infected. Although most babies will initially test positive for their mothers' HIV antibodies, only 15 to 30 percent are actually infected with the disease. Children may also be infected through breast-feeding.

In 1994, the CDC issued new recommendations for preventing HIV transmission from pregnant women to their babies by beginning treatment with zidovudine (AZT) during the early stages of pregnancy. Research has shown that, for HIV-positive women who were treated with a daily regimen of this drug during pregnancy and delivery and whose babies were treated with the drug after birth, only 8.3 percent of the infants were infected with HIV disease, compared with 25 percent of those born to untreated women. AZT treatment also did not appear to have adverse effects on the health of the pregnant women, although the CDC recommends that all mothers and children receive long-term follow-up care since long-term effects of the treatment are unknown.

This powerful advance in reducing the risk of prenatal AIDS has given new hope to many HIV-positive women who wish to have children. An HIV-positive woman still has to decide to take the risk of exposing a child to HIV infection, although the risk is smaller. She also must decide whether to have a child that may be left motherless, as she will probably die before the child reaches adulthood. Estimates are that by the year 2000, more than 80,000 children will be motherless as a result of AIDS. Women also must make choices about breast-feeding because it is a known route of transmission of HIV to an infant, and AZT treatment may not prevent transmission.

Counselors can help clients decide whether to take these risks. To be sensitive to a woman's concerns, counselors must be aware of the influence of various cultural values about motherhood on women from different backgrounds. For some women, childbearing may be seen as a religious or family duty. In some cultures, the ability to bear a child may be a source of pride for a woman and a proof of manliness for her partner.

Many women may react negatively to a counseling approach that assumes that the only choice for women who are HIV-positive is to forego having children. Instead, a counselor may inform a woman of the risks of infecting her children and discuss options that help a woman make informed decisions about pregnancy, childbirth, and breast-feeding. Discussion of risks should recognize the family and social environment of each woman. It may be helpful to find an HIV-positive woman who has already made similar decisions to talk with a client. Clients may be referred to health centers that can give them more complete information about medical risks and treatments.

Promoting Preventive Behaviors for Women at Risk for HIV

Psychological and Social Factors

Many women who are at high-risk appear to be unresponsive to preventive intervention. Prevention programs must take into account the factors that impede the process of behavior change that would reduce women's HIV risk. Programs for women must do much more than instruct women in the use of condoms. Risk reduction programs must be responsive to the social context in which women make decisions. The following list shows some of the psychological and social barriers to the adoption of preventive behaviors that CMHC staff will need to consider.

Psychological and Social Barriers to the Adoption of Preventive Behaviors

- Fear of violence
- Emphasis on maintaining relationships
- Economic dependence
- Self-esteem that is tied to traditional gender roles
- Lack of social support

Fear of Violence

Violence against women is frequent in our society. Many women live in situations in which they are physically or sexually abused. Many young women who use drugs are running away from unsafe, violent families. Prevention workers have learned that it is not simple for women who fear violence to initiate discussions of safer sex or to adopt new, safer practices. For example, outreach programs for women in the sex trade found that women would demand the use of condoms with customers, but not from their pimps, either out of fear or from a desire to please the person with whom they had a primary relationship. Women who are in relationships with abusive men or who are financially dependent upon their partners may be unable to initiate new behavior. Women may experience more domestic violence while they are pregnant (Rothenberg and Paskey, 1995). Because women often learn their HIV status during pregnancy, their risk of physical abuse may increase during this time.

Importance of Relationships with Others

Women's social training about the meaning of relationships in their lives makes it difficult to challenge the attitudes or behaviors of their partners which place them at risk for HIV. Women who have been trained to be "other-directed" may put so much importance on maintaining their relationships with men, or, if lesbian, with other women, that they will risk contracting HIV rather than strain their relationship.

A woman's need for approval will influence her decisions about HIV prevention. She may be reluctant to ask questions about her partner's sexual or drug use behavior or to insist on safer practices. Women's reasons for having sex vary. These reasons include sex for intimacy, acceptance, duty, pleasure, money, or protection. Women may continue to have unsafe sex for fear of abandonment, rejection, or violence. A woman may be ambivalent about her rights in a relationship. Women in traditional sex role relationships may believe that it is not right to challenge men's rights in marriage. Some women believe that sex is a duty to their partners. Some women believe that you should do anything for someone you love.

Economic Dependence

Many women who are most vulnerable to HIV infection are dependent upon men for economic support. This dependency often determines whether a woman may demand safety for herself. Her choice may be between protected sex or continued financial support. Women who are dependent upon men for drugs or the money to purchase drugs may forego safer sex in exchange for what they need.

Self-esteem

Many women who engage in behaviors that place them at high risk for HIV may not perceive themselves in danger. If a woman lacks a sense of self-worth or feels hopeless about her situation, her only coping strategy may be to deny personal vulnerability to HIV. In our culture, a woman's self-esteem is often based on her ability to fulfill the traditional roles of sexual partner and child bearer. HIV disease threatens both of those roles. Society, as well as the family, may devalue a woman who cannot safely bear more children or who continues to bear children who are at risk of being born HIV-infected. Being less desirable sexually can be very threatening to women. It may be so threatening that some women may not disclose their HIV status or may continue to practice unsafe sex for fear of alienating a male partner.

Lack of Social Support

Many HIV-positive women, especially those who use drugs, have very few social supports. Women may be rejected by partners or family members and friends after they disclose their status. Many women who take care of partners with AIDS may not have a network of people who will, in turn, take care of them when they become sick.

Strategies for Prevention for Women

HIV prevention programs for women must be based on changes in life-style which women must make to protect themselves. Research shows that a woman's ability to implement health education messages depends upon self-esteem, a sense of personal power and her interpretation of gender roles, as well as her education and socioeconomic status. Changes in life-style often require a fundamental reorganization of a woman's life. Social support to make and maintain such changes is important. Many women who are vulnerable to HIV disease will overcome barriers to change more easily if prevention programs recognize and provide some of the necessary supports.

Prevention Strategies for Women at Risk

- Design programs that promote self-care.
- Include the entire family as the focus for prevention.
- Develop woman-focused methods for safer sex.
- Focus prevention messages on culturally relevant communications between women and their sexual partners.

- Provide safe environments for women to discuss sexual issues.
- Assess the risk of violence and offer interventions.
- Pursue aggressive outreach to women who use drugs.
- Advocate for support services such as:

    –Multi-service, well-woman clinics;

    –Child care respite programs;

    –Nutrition supplements for women and their children;

    –Low cost, neighborhood health programs.

Promoting Good Self-care

Cultural barriers to good self-care for women limit the success of health prevention programs. These barriers include value systems that teach women to consider everyone else's welfare before their own. Women are still the caretakers in our culture and often receive little support for taking care of themselves. Care of others before oneself has been taught as part of a woman's role as a good daughter, wife, and mother. Women often deprive themselves, with pride, in order to provide food, clothing, and medical care for their children. Focusing on self is often seen by society as selfish rather than as evidence of good self-esteem. Women are still rewarded socially in many cultures for postponing their own dreams in favor of their husband's and children's dreams.

Prevention programs must address these values on community and family levels rather than only on individual levels. For women to "put their own welfare first" requires finding ways for women to be rewarded socially for other things rather than becoming martyrs for their families. Families or partners may sabotage women's efforts to change, particularly if the changes are perceived as threats to traditional sex role divisions. For example, research indicates that men in our society still resist assuming equal care of home and children, particularly for tasks considered traditionally to be "women's work." Women who attempt to introduce changes in sexual practices may be viewed as directly threatening men's vested roles in the family.

Good self-care includes medical care, healthy nutrition, rest, and avoidance of stress. For poor or low-income women, these conditions are sometimes impossible to achieve. Prevention programs must acknowledge the real conditions of women's lives and work within these realities to achieve change. CMHC staff may need to become advocates for the development of programs for women that go beyond education. Well-women clinics, child-care respite programs, nutrition supplement programs, free or low-cost neighborhood health programs, and community programs that promote and reinforce new social norms that benefit women are possible ways to help women achieve better care.

Woman-Focused Preventive Education

Understanding sex role beliefs and the rights and duties in relationships held by women and men of different socioeconomic, cultural, and ethnic backgrounds is important for the CMHC clinician. As the AIDS epidemic continues, more women will be seropositive and asymptomatic for a longer number of years. Women need information on how to limit re-exposure to HIV, as well as more methods that will allow them to lead normal sex lives. A number of women have urged that funding be made available for more development and testing of products that women may use to protect themselves and that they can control, such as vaginal sponges, condoms for women, and viricidal solutions. Early research showed that women respond positively to the new female condoms, but more research is needed on their effectiveness and women's willingness to use them consistently.

Most successful safer sex prevention programs have focused on developing strategies that empower women and improve their ability to advocate for their needs. Education programs stress skill development in discussing sex with men. Role-playing of social interactions in which women formulate options and practice their repertoires are used frequently. More strategies are needed for helping women and men discuss sexual practices directly. Prevention workers have also recognized the importance of aggressive outreach efforts directed at both women and their partners. Some programs focus on taking the burden of change from women by emphasizing the need for men to change sexual practices. Efforts directed at reaching women include social programs that provide direct, visible services for high-risk or HIV-positive women. These programs must be culturally relevant to the target populations.

Women with HIV disease will be able to make only changes that do not increase the risk of violence from partners. Counseling should include an assessment of the risk of domestic violence and referrals to community programs that can help a woman reduce her risk. Many health agencies do not routinely ask questions about women's injuries or the extent to which women suffer emotional and/or physical abuse. Counselors and physicians should probably accept a woman's report of fear as a real risk and refrain from any actions that would increase her risk of violence from a partner.

Aggressive Outreach to Women Who Use Drugs

Since drug use, and sex with men who use drugs, are the most prevalent modes of transmission of HIV for women, prevention must focus on reaching women who are part of the drug culture. Access to drug treatment and rehabilitation programs is an essential part of prevention to reduce the craving for drugs that overcomes good judgment about safer sex practices. More drug treatment opportunities for women, especially for pregnant women and mothers of small children, are needed to increase the chances for behavioral treatment programs to work once a woman is in recovery. For women who trade or sell sex for drugs, risk reduction programs are needed that are integrated with mental health services and drug treatment.

Studies have shown that community programs can reach women whose partners are HIV-positive. The most effective models appear to be aggressive outreach programs that use prevention workers of the same racial or ethnic background who are in recovery from drug addiction to recruit women into self-help programs. Community mental health centers can be on the front lines of drug rehabilitation programs, using these models in the hiring and training of community outreach workers and drug counselors. Programs must exhibit concern for the well-being of women as valuable people and must be based on empowering women to obtain the resources they need to reinforce sobriety and self-protection.

Helping Women with HIV Disease to Access Appropriate Medical and Mental Healthcare

Services for Women with HIV Disease

- Routine HIV risk assessment for women and their children during intake interviews
- Day care for uninfected children while mothers and any children with HIV in the family receive medical or mental health treatment
- Mental healthcare that is sensitive to a woman's cultural belief system
- Expanded drug treatment programs for women that provide:
    - –Child care
    - –Job training
    - –Housing during recovery
- HIV support groups for women
- Assistance in locating basic resources
- Participation in interagency case coordination

Mental health counselors must assume that clients are at risk and include HIV risk assessments as part of intake interviews. Be prepared to make appropriate referrals for HIV counseling and testing. Assess the service needs of women as well as their children. Women who are HIV-positive may have one or more children with the disease who also need services. They may also have uninfected children who are affected by the illness of their mother and siblings. Many programs are finding that day care for siblings who are not infected is an important component of the mother's physical and mental healthcare. The entire family unit is affected when a mother is ill. A mother, her children, partner or spouse, and the extended family will all have concerns about how HIV will affect their family.

Assessing Family and Social Support

In our culture, it is still more acceptable for women to be other-directed than to focus on themselves. Even when women with HIV disease are ill, their functions as caretakers of others remain at the forefront of their concerns. Family members often assume that women will continue to look after other people and will not require corresponding care for themselves. Approaches that place women first may fail both with the client and within her family.

An assessment can ascertain the belief system operating in a family and the patterns of caretaking to determine how the woman's needs are being met. Some health centers report that it is easier to bring women into social and medical care systems if their children are the primary focus of care. Approaches that suggest that only if a mother takes proper care of herself will her children be secure may be more effective than appeals that she consider her own health.

Locating and Negotiating Family-Centered Care

HIV medical care clinics and CMHCs can be organized to provide care for adult women with HIV and any of their children who are HIV-positive, and psychosocial services for uninfected siblings. Day care should be provided while the women and their children are waiting for treatment or while the mothers consult healthcare providers. Such a multiservice approach also minimizes the expense of traveling to various clinics. Some cities are organizing these multiservice centers through cooperating agencies that rotate staff to these centers.

Finding Drug Addiction Treatment Programs

Social service workers have pointed out that the number of drug treatment facilities and beds in inpatient clinics are proportionally less for women than for men. More outpatient treatment programs are needed. Treatment programs must help women with child care arrangements during treatment and with job skills and housing as part of the recovery process. Studies of chemically dependent women show that most women in federally funded drug treatment programs lack a high school education and are unemployed. Many women will not enter treatment programs because the programs do not provide child care and they risk losing their children to foster care.

Special outreach for the non-drug-using female partners of injecting drug users is needed. These women are still a hidden population who can benefit from programs designed to address their needs.

Providing Support Groups

Support groups for women with HIV are becoming more common. The value of these woman-only groups is that they enable women with HIV to overcome some of the isolation and stigma of having the disease. Women who are HIV-positive may never have met another woman with the disease. Most support groups have been organized for men. Women may feel outnumbered in such groups or feel embarrassed about discussing some aspects of their diseases.

Community mental health centers may provide special groups for women who have been isolated from others with similar problems. Women who are recovering from drug use, women with children, lesbians, bisexual women, and women who contracted HIV disease from sex with bisexual men or men who use drugs are groups that might benefit from a safe, accepting environment in which to discuss issues that are unique to them.

Conclusion

As the HIV epidemic spreads, there is some indication that women will become the most at risk group for HIV infection. CMHC staff must focus on how to counsel and support women who are suffering as individuals, rather than simply as people who may place children and men at risk. Services are needed that are woman-focused and that begin from the point of view of the women served. Community mental health centers, with their tradition of client-focused community services, have a unique opportunity and responsibility to provide leadership for community HIV services for women. Community mental health centers can strengthen their ability to serve women by being sensitive to all populations at risk. They can provide consultation to primary medical care facilities in the community to help develop sensitive protocols for women's care. Much of the work of CMHC staff will be to establish referral mechanisms and participate in interagency case coordination efforts. Serving women with HIV requires extensive interagency coordination. Women with HIV disease need assistance with mental healthcare, medical care, nutrition, finances, housing, employment, transportation, child care, legal assistance, and negotiating the many agencies that provide these services.

Review Questions

1. What are clients conveying about the way discrimination affects their lives? What do you observe?

2. What kinds of changes are needed in community mental health programs that would alleviate discrimination that affects women?

3. How can counselors and medical providers be more responsive to women who use drugs or who are partners of people who use drugs?

4. How can mental healthcare providers help women who are HIV-positive to find adequate healthcare?

References and Suggested Readings

Buehler, J.W., Ward, J.W., & Berelman, R.L. (1993). The surveillance definition for AIDS in the United States. *AIDS, 7,* 585–587.

Carpenter, C.C., Mayer, K.H., Stein, M.D., Leibman, B.D., Fisher, A., & Fiore, T.C. (1991). Human immunodeficiency virus infection in North American women: Experience with 200 cases and a review of the literature. *Medicine, 70*(5), 307–325.

Centers for Disease Control and Prevention. (1997). *HIV/AIDS Surveillance Report, 8*(2).

Centers for Disease Control and Prevention. (1994). Zidovudine for the prevention of HIV transmission from mother to infant. *Mortality and Morbidity Weekly Report, 43,* 285–287.

Chung, J.Y., & Magraw, M.M. (1992). A group approach to psychosocial issues faced by HIV-positive women. *Hospital and Community Psychiatry, 43*(9), 891–894.

Cochran, S.D. (1989). Women and HIV infection. In V. Mays, G.W. Albee, & S.F. Schneider (Eds.). *Primary Prevention of AIDS: Psychological Approaches.* Newbury Park, CA: Sage Publications.

Coodley, G.O., Coodley, M.K., & Thompson, A.F. (1995). Clinical aspects of HIV infection in women. *Journal of General Internal Medicine, 10*(2), 99–110.

Cooper, E.B. (1995). Historical and analytical overview of policy issues affecting women living with AIDS: A blueprint for learning from our past. *Bulletin of the New York Academy of Medicine, 72*(suppl 1), 283–299.

DeSantis, M., Noia, G., Caruso, A., & Mancuso, S. (1995). Guidelines for the use of Zidovudine in pregnant women with HIV infection. *Drugs, 50*(1), 43–47.

Dickover, R.E., Garratty, E.M., Herman, S.A., Sim, M.S., Plaeger, S., Boyer, P.J., Keller, M., Deveikis, A., Stiehm, E.R., & Bryson, Y.J. (1996). Identification of levels of maternal HIV-1 RNA associated with risk of perinatal transmission: Effect of maternal zidovudine treatment on viral load. *Journal of the American Medical Association, 275*(8), 599–605.

Ehrhardt, A., Exner, T., & Seal, D.W. (1997). A review of HIV interventions for at-risk women. In

Office of Technology Assessment. (1997). *The Effectiveness of AIDS Prevention Efforts: A State of the Science Report.* Washington, D.C.: American Psychological Association Office on AIDS.

El-Bassel, N., Schilling, R.F., Irwin, K.L., Faruque, S., Gilbert, L., Von Bargen, J., Serrano, Y., & Edlin, B.R. (1997). Sex trading and psychological distress among women recruited from the streets of Harlem. *American Journal of Public Health, 87*(1), 66–70.

Goldsmith, M.F. (1992). Specific HIV-related problems of women gain more attention at a price—affecting more women. *Journal of the American Medical Association, 268*(14), 1814–1816.

Gollub, E.L., Stein, Z., & El-Sader, W. (1995). Short-term acceptability of the female condom among staff and patients at a New York City hospital. *Family Planning and Perspectives, 27*(4), 155–158.

Guinan, M.E., & Leviton, L. (1995). Prevention of HIV infection in women: Overcoming barriers. *Journal of the American Medical Women Association, 50*(3–4), 74–77.

Heckman, T.G., Sikkema, K.J., Kelly, J.A., Fuqua, R.W., Mercer, M.B., Hoffmann, R.G., Winett, R.A., Anderson, E.S., Perry, M.J., Roffman, R.A., Solomon, L.J., Wagstaff, D.A., Cargill, V., Norman, A.D., & Crumble, D. (1996). Predictors of condom use and human immunodeficiency virus test seeking among women living in inner-city public housing developments. *Sexually Transmitted Diseases, 23*(5), 357–365.

Hillemans, P., Ellerbrock, T.V., McPhillips, S., Dole, P., Alperstein, S., Johnson, D., Sun, X.W., Chiasson, M.A., & Wright, T.C., Jr. (1996). Prevalence of anal human *Papillomavirus* infection and anal cytologic abnormalities in HIV-seropositive women. *AIDS, 10*(14), 1641–1647.

Holtgrave, D.R., & Kelly, J.A. (1996). Preventing HIV/AIDS among high-risk women: The cost-effectiveness of a behavioral group intervention. *American Journal of Public Health, 86*(10), 1442–1445.

Kass, N.E. (1994). Policy, ethics, and reproductive choice: Pregnancy and childbearing among HIV-infected women. *Acta Pædiatrica Supplement, 400*, 95–98.

Kennedy, M.B., Scarlett, M.I., Duerr, A.C., & Chu, S.Y. (1995). Assessing HIV risk among women who have sex with women: Scientific and communication issues. *Journal of the American Women Association, 50*(304), 103–107.

Kissinger, P., Clark, R., Dumestre, J., & Bessinger, R. (1996). Incidence of three sexually transmitted diseases during a safer sex promotion program for HIV-infected women. *Journal of General Internal Medicine, 11*(12), 750–752.

Korn, A.P., & Landers, D.V. (1995). Gynecologic disease in women infected with human immunodeficiency virus type 1. *Journal of Acquired Immune Deficiency Syndromes and Human Retrovirology, 9*(4), 361–370.

Michaels D., & Levine C. (1992). Estimates of the number of motherless youth orphaned by AIDS in the United States. *Journal of the American Medical Association, 268*, 3456–3461.

Minkoff, H.L., & DeHovitz, J.A. (1991). Care of women infected with the human immunodeficiency virus. *Journal of the American Medical Association, 266*(16), 2253–2258.

Mondanaro, J. (1989). *Chemically Dependent Women.* Lexington, MA: Lexington Books.

Pearlberg, G. (1991). *Women, AIDS and Communities: A Guide for Action.* Metuchen, NJ: Women's Action Alliance and Scarecrow Press.

Person, B., & Cotton, D. (1996). A model of community mobilization for the prevention of HIV in women and infants. *Public Health Reports, 111*(suppl 1), 89–98.

Rothenberg, K.H., & Paskey, S.J. (1995). The risk of domestic violence and women with HIV infection: Implications for partner notification, public policy, and the law. *American Journal of Public Health, 85*(11), 1569–1576.

Shervington, D.O. (1993). The acceptability of the female condom among low-income African-American women. *Journal of the National Medical Association, 85,* 341–347.

Shotsky, W.J. (1996). Women who have sex with other women: HIV seroprevalence in New York State counseling and testing programs. *Women's Health, 24*(2), 1–15.

Simpson, B.J., Shapiro, E.D., and Andiman, W.A. (1997). Reduction in the Risk of Vertical Transmission of HIV-1 Associated with Treatment of Pregnant Women with Orally Administered Lidovirdine Alone. *Journal of AIDS & Human Retrovirology, 14*(2), 145–152.

U.S. Congress. (1990). *Beyond the Stereotypes: Women, Addiction and Perinatal Substance Abuse.* Hearing before the House Select Committee on Children, Youth and Families. 101st Congress, Second Session, April 19, 1990. Washington, D.C.: Government Printing Office.

U.S. Congress. (1992). *Women and HIV Disease: Falling Through the Cracks.* Hearing before the House Committee on Governmental Operations; Human Resources and Intergovernmental Relations Subcommittee. 102nd Congress, First Session, June 6, 1991. Washington, D.C.: Government Printing Office.

Watstein, S., & Laurich, R.A. (1991). *AIDS and Women: A Sourcebook.* Phoenix, AZ: Oryx Press.

Wermuth, L., Ham, J., & Robbins, R. (1992). Women don't wear condoms: AIDS risk among sexual partners of IV drug users. In J. Huber & B. Schneider (Eds.), *The Social Context of AIDS.* Newbury Park, CA: Sage Publications.

Wingood, G.M., & DiClemente, R.J. (1996). HIV sexual risk redution interventions for women: A review. *American Journal of Preventive Medicine, 12*(3), 209–217.

Worth, D. (1990). Minority women and AIDS: Culture, race and gender. In D.A. Feldman (Ed.), *Culture and AIDS.* New York: Praeger.

Zierler, S., Witbeck, B., & Mayer, K. (1996). Sexual violence against women living with or at risk for HIV infection. *American Journal of Preventive Medicine, 12*(5), 304–310.

Chapter 16

Multicultural Issues in Treating African-Americans and Latinos

Derise E. Tolliver, Ph.D.,
José A. Parés-Avila, M.A.,
Rubén Montano-López, M.A., and
Nicolás P. Carballeira, N.D., M.P.H.

Overview

This chapter is designed to help community mental health center (CMHC) clinicians provide culturally competent services to African-Americans and Latinos with HIV/AIDS. The goal is to familiarize clinicians with important cultural and cross-cultural issues to promote more sensitive assessment, counseling, and referral of HIV-infected members of these populations and their families.

Learning Objectives

1. To recognize the cross-cultural response continuum and the basic requirements of cross-cultural competence in delivering mental health services.

2. To develop knowledge of the diversity among persons with HIV/AIDS in the African-American and Latino communities, the characteristics of the HIV epidemic in these populations, and those commonly shared values that may serve as a context for a mental health intervention.

3. To describe at least four strategies that overcome linguistic and cultural barriers, and at the same time respect and incorporate commonly shared values in the provision of services.

Outline

   I. The Cross-Cultural Response

     A. Response continuum: destructiveness to competence

     B. Client reactions

     C. Requirements of cross-cultural competence

  II. Minorities and HIV/AIDS

 III. African-Americans and HIV/AIDS

     A. Issues in interventions with HIV-infected African-American clients

        1. Attitudes toward homosexuality

        2. Attitudes toward drug use

        3. Influence of culture and religion on discussion of sexuality

     B. Working with families

     C. Women's issues

     D. Using cultural strengths

     E. The need for self-assessment

 IV. Latinos and HIV/AIDS

     A. Transmission of HIV among Latinos

     B. Considerations and strategies for effective interventions with clients from the Latino population

        1. Country of origin

        2. Language use

        3. Natural support systems

        4. Other considerations

The Cross-Cultural Response

Counseling people living with HIV/AIDS presents new challenges to CMHC clinicians, particularly since the service population is drawn from multiple cultures.

Although there are excellent materials and resources available about the clinical and scientific aspects of HIV/AIDS, there is less information and assistance regarding counseling persons from diverse cultural backgrounds.

Mental health providers are often unaware of basic principles of cross-cultural service delivery, including the definition and significance of culture as a factor in counseling, the dominant cultural values common to specific patient populations, and the ways in which the dominant provider culture influences the delivery of services and the attitudes toward persons living with HIV/AIDS.

This chapter is intended to familiarize the community mental health worker with some of the cultural issues that will promote more sensitive screening, counseling, and referrals for clients from African-American and Latino populations. Professionals who are members of these two communities have collaborated as authors of this chapter.

Response Continuum: Destructiveness to Competence

Whenever a provider and a client from different cultures meet, there are potential barriers to service delivery. It is important that CMHC staff examine ways in which their cultural behavior may influence the degree of acculturation exhibited by a client.

A model of cross-cultural responses and levels of acculturation is useful for understanding the range of responses that can take place between mental health provider and client. Responses may range from destructiveness to cultural competence on the part of the provider with client responses ranging from resistance to biculturality. In our society, the healthcare provider usually controls important aspects of the therapeutic relationship, including site, environment, time of initiation, duration, and type of intervention. The provider controls the cross-cultural tone of the relationship. Possible provider cross-cultural behavior includes: destructiveness, incapacity, blindness, sensitivity, and competence.

Destructiveness

The provider considers the client's culture inferior or worthless and actively tries to impose his or her values and world view. The intervention attempts to discount the client's values and replace them as a precondition for a therapeutic relationship.

Incapacity

The provider acknowledges cultural differences but has no skills or tools to address them effectively and therefore proceeds with a standard intervention based on dominant cultural values. As a cross-cultural response, incapacity may be a long-term approach to multiculturality.

Blindness

The provider considers that all humans share basic values and therefore treats all people alike, regardless of their differences. Such behavior is culture-bound, culture-blind, for all its apparent universality, and results in a standard intervention based on the cultural values of the provider.

Sensitivity

The provider acknowledges differences and tries to address them by adopting external or formal cultural expressions and presenting the standard intervention within these parameters. Cultural sensitivity usually is limited to the use of the client's language and literacy level, and respect for major, obvious taboos.

Competence

The provider identifies, respects, and incorporates the values of the client in the design, delivery, and evaluation of the service. The intervention is client-centered; the provider listens actively, elicits the client's world view, acknowledges the differences and similarities, recommends approaches congruent with the client's values, and negotiates their implementation or adaptation.

Client Reactions

Faced with one of these cultural responses, a client from a nondominant culture might exhibit one of the following reactions: resistance, assimilation, or biculturality.

Resistance

The client refuses to participate in the intervention, is unresponsive, and may exhibit either hostility or passivity. Often in the Latino community, for example, the client will purposely minimize his or her understanding of the English language.

Assimilation

The client rejects his or her native culture and attempts to adopt the values, attitudes, and behavior that he or she perceives to be dominant. The client tries to please the provider and agrees to recommendations that are impractical or inappropriate.

Biculturality

The client maintains his or her values, attitudes, and behaviors, adapting them to new circumstances, while simultaneously adopting skills and strategies that allow him or her to function effectively within the dominant culture.

Cross-cultural Response	Client Reaction
■ Destructiveness	Resistance
	Assimilation
■ Incapacity	Resistance
	Assimilation
■ Blindness	Resistance
	Assimilation
■ Sensitivity	Resistance
	Assimilation
	Biculturality
■ Competence	Biculturality

The preceding table identifies some cross-cultural responses and client reactions that are most probable within their context. Cultural destructiveness allows for a response of either resistance or assimilation but will, generally, elicit only the latter since the client is in a dependent role. It may seem too dangerous to respond otherwise in the face of a counselor who demonstrates destructive responses to a client's cultural values and experience. Incapacity and blindness often are met with resistance or assimilation.

Cultural sensitivity on the part of a provider is met by clients with the entire spectrum of acculturation. When the intervention is too superficially "sensitive" it will appear disingenuous, and clients may respond with passive resistance. More commonly, clients accept the sensitive aspects of the intervention and reject the core, which is based on the provider's cultural values.

Cultural competence alone encourages and accepts biculturality in clients; it openly recognizes and respects the differences and similarities in world view, while incorporating the client's values in the service core.

Requirements of Cross-cultural Competence

The context of mental health interventions is not neutral. People bring their power or lack of it to their interactions with providers, and providers bring their values, attitudes, and professional behavior into the equation. "Professional" implies standard beliefs and behavior. HIV infection makes the connection between cultural powerlessness and disease obvious and inescapable. At its most basic level, AIDS is the lack of power to resist disease.

This culturally driven biological powerlessness is part of a pattern that also manifests itself as social, economic, political, and emotional disempowerment. When we add a cross-cultural encounter to this already charged situation, the probability of an effective mental health intervention is diminished if the provider is unable to adequately adapt to the changing demands of diverse client populations and of each specific client.

An effective approach to cross-cultural HIV/AIDS counseling is one that breaks the pattern of powerlessness by eliciting from the client those values that are deeply held and bases the intervention on those values. Providers can then produce congruent behaviors, attitudes, and practices that enable them to address the concerns of their clients within a shared context.

Minorities and HIV/AIDS

As of December 1996, there had been 581,429 AIDS cases reported in the United States, its commonwealths, and territories. It is estimated that more than a hundred people die of AIDS in the United States every day. Cumulative cases reported to the Centers for Disease Control and Prevention as of the end of December, 1996 included 203,189 cases among African-Americans (35% of the total) and 103,023 among Latinos (18% of the total). This compares with 268,856 (46%) for Caucasians.

In spite of the continuing misconceptions about AIDS being a disease of gay white men, the statistics clearly indicate that AIDS cases are increasing among the two largest minority populations represented in the following illustration.

In 1996, African-Americans, who constitute only 12 percent of the U.S. population, accounted for 35 percent of all reported AIDS cases. They also accounted for disproportionate numbers in all categories of people with AIDS, including heterosexual men, women, and children. Once exposed to the virus, African-Americans progress more quickly to the final stage of HIV disease, and they have a shorter life expectancy once diagnosed with AIDS than do Caucasians. This is at least partly the result of late diagnosis and inadequate medical care.

Cumulative AIDS Cases in the U.S. African-American Population, through December 1996

- In December 1996, 12% of the U.S. population was African-American.
- 35% of all reported AIDS cases were African-Americans.
- 31% of men with AIDS are African-American.
- 55% of women with AIDS are African-American.

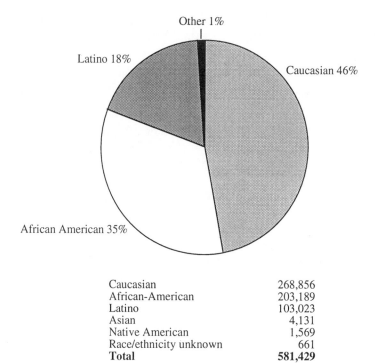

Caucasian	268,856
African-American	203,189
Latino	103,023
Asian	4,131
Native American	1,569
Race/ethnicity unknown	661
Total	**581,429**

FIGURE 16.1 Cumulative U.S. AIDS cases by race/ethnicity, through December 1996.

■ 58% of children with AIDS are African-American.

■ 39% of African-Americans with AIDS are injecting drug users.

■ 52% of African-American children with AIDS are born to mothers who were injecting drug users or partners of injecting drug users.

The relative risk of AIDS for Latinos seems to be much higher in the north-eastern United States and Puerto Rico. AIDS cases reported in Puerto Rico alone represent over 18 percent of the total Latino AIDS cases in the United States. Recent statistics from the Puerto Rico Health Department show that AIDS is already the leading cause of death for men 30 to 39 years of age and for women between the ages of 25 to 29 years.

African-Americans and HIV/AIDS

CMHC staff who work with African-American clients need to understand their culture and psychology. Being African-American in a society where racism and discrimination exist affects healthcare, health status, and quality of life, which in turn influence the course of HIV disease. In addition, race and cultural values influence attitudes, beliefs, and behavior regarding health and illness, help-seeking, sexuality, and drug use—all relevant concerns of counseling. When working with African-American clients, it is important to begin with an understanding of how they assess their own needs.

Issues in Interventions with HIV-Infected African-American Clients

Overall Counseling Approach with African-American Clients

- Identify and work with the client's own assessment of his or her problems and needs.
- Use a concrete, problem-solving counseling approach to address the most immediate survival concerns.
- Support behavior change through role-playing, skill-building activities, and support groups.
- Do not force the client to focus on intrapsychic, talk-oriented counseling before he or she is ready.
- Build rapport by relating to the client as a respected and valuable person.

A concrete, problem-solving counseling approach has been reported to best help African-American clients address their most immediate survival concerns associated with AIDS, including housing, medical care, and employment. Counseling sessions should also include education on risk-reduction activities. Counselors can support client behavior change through role playing, skill-building activities, and support groups. These approaches, which are active and social in nature, are consistent with an African-American-centered style of relating and instruction. Success in these areas can foster increased trust in the counselor and a willingness on the client's part to eventually engage in talk-oriented, insight work.

Specific Approaches for Intervention with African-American Clients

- Be willing to "chat" with the client to further develop trust and build rapport.
- Be clear about confidentiality—clarify what information has to be shared and which information the client wants to share with others.

- Accept the client's comfort level in talking about feelings.

- Use Black English vernacular only if you feel comfortable with this and can do so in a way that does not seem artificial.

- Focus on the need for the client to change high-risk behavior rather than labeling client as a member of a disfavored group (e.g., gay, drug user).

- Appeal to the client's responsibility and concern for children and family as reasons for behavior change.

- With African-American women, provide counseling on self-esteem and self-empowerment, as well as education and skill-building activities.

- Use cultural strengths to help African-American clients more successfully deal with AIDS.

African-Americans are often suspicious of counselors from a different cultural background and of those who approach the work as strictly business. Often, a client will ask personal questions about the counselor's marital status, place of residence, and other personal issues as a way of establishing "equality" in the relationship. What may seem to be unprofessional and unnecessary self-disclosure to a CMHC staff person may be very important to the client in her or his effort to determine whether to trust a staff member. A counselor should expect to chat during some initial sessions and understand that this may be necessary to develop trust and rapport.

Because high-risk behavior and a diagnosis of HIV disease or AIDS may jeopardize many aspects of their lives, most African-American clients are concerned about who will have access to the information that they share with the counselor. It is important for counselors to be candid from the very beginning about accessibility of clients' statements and records. Counselors should also clarify what information the client wishes to share with whom. It is imperative that individual counselors and CMHC workers review record keeping and other operations to make sure that confidentiality is not inadvertently breached because of institutionalized procedures as when, for example, all AIDS patients are seen on a certain day by a certain clinician.

Counselors must also be aware that their expectations about communication may differ from that of their African-American clients. Clients may not feel comfortable talking directly about their feelings, but rather assume that feelings are evident through their nonverbal expressiveness. They may feel the need to control their emotions or not share feelings that would be embarrassing. It is most important to "listen" to what the client does as well as says. The counselor can acknowledge the client's discomfort, as well as possible distrust, of the counseling process. This may help to validate the client's experience.

Some people think that the counselor must use scientific terms to discuss taboo subjects such as sexuality and drug abuse, but this is not so. It is important to learn, understand, and respect the beliefs and the language that the client uses. It is not necessary to "force" clients to use the "correct" technical language if by using their own language they better understand what the counselor is trying to communicate. Some clients will be more comfortable with the use of "street" terms. However, workers should not use Black English vernacular or any language pattern that does not feel comfortable to them. To do so will likely be seen as phony and nonauthentic by the client.

Counselors may misinterpret communication styles of African-American clients. For example, African-Americans are often labeled as inappropriately angry and hostile. However, their experiences with racism and discrimination in our society have left many of them feeling powerless, alienated, and angry. Similarly, the experience of AIDS leaves many clients angry because of the profound changes it produces in their lives. It is important for the CMHC counselor to help the client distinguish between anger resulting from present or past difficulties, and to address it accordingly.

Attitudes toward Homosexuality

Homosexuality has been shrouded in secrecy within the African-American community. As with most communities of color, it has long been considered a taboo that is neither openly nor easily discussed. Major institutions, such as churches, have actively disapproved of this sexual orientation. Therefore, the experience of being gay in the African-American community is often punctuated by dilemmas and difficulties. If one is gay, and facing HIV/AIDS, the stress of keeping secrets, deciding who to inform not only of one's HIV status but perhaps also of one's life-style, and the possible consequences of such disclosure may be some of the issues that are brought to therapy. To be most effective, it is important for the CMHC counselor to be aware of the cultural context in which the gay African-American client lives.

The pressure to conform to group norms, the importance of the family, and the desire to maintain status and approval within the community results in some African-American men marrying and having children while maintaining sexual relationships with other men. They may not consider themselves bisexual or gay. Similarly, unmarried men out of fear of rejection by the community may not have revealed that they are gay or bisexual. Consequently, it may be more important for the CMHC counselor to appeal to a man's sense of responsibility to himself, his family, and cultural community, and to focus on specific behavior, rather than to ask about an identity that the client may not embrace. This approach will also be useful for those gay and bisexual African-American clients who are not questioning nor in distress about their sexual orientation.

Attitudes toward Drug Use

Injection drug use is a primary risk factor for HIV transmission in the African-American community. In addition to the hazards of sharing needles and drug paraphernalia, drug use becomes a bridge for the infection of women who may be sexual partners of injecting drug users. Women, in turn, may transmit the virus to their unborn children. Because of social and legal prohibitions, drug users may be reluctant to discuss their practices openly and may require additional assurance of acceptance and confidentiality. Counselors should describe the danger of sharing needles, methods of cleaning needles and works, and safer sex practices. They should also encourage clients to enter substance abuse programs and actively advocate on their behalf for effective treatment.

Influence of Culture and Religion on Discussion of Sexuality

For some African-American clients, cultural and religious values dictate whether they can discuss matters of sexuality with someone outside the family or with a stranger. If there are religious sanctions against sex for other than procreative purposes, clients may need support and guidance to deal with these as well as AIDS issues. It may help to refer them to community resources affiliated with their own religion.

Working with Families

Family is very important in the African-American community and will probably be a focus in AIDS-related work with African-American clients. Often, client concerns center on informing family members about the AIDS diagnosis and associated high-risk behavior, how to deal with absence of family support and understanding, and how to obtain needed support. The counselor can help the client decide how and to whom to disclose their HIV status using role-playing and rehearsal.

By working with the family and providing the latest accurate information, the counselor can help minimize the stigma of AIDS and prepare the client and family to get the support that will be needed. Adult clients with AIDS may be returning to their parents' home after having lived independently, and this may place additional tensions on the family, especially if there already were conflicts about the client's life-style. Family counseling and support groups should be made available to help the primarily female caregivers cope with the stress accompanying their role.

Women's Issues

Many heterosexual African-American women are in situations where they perceive themselves to be powerless to demand HIV risk-reduction behavior from their sexual partners. They may be financially or emotionally dependent upon their partner and fear that insisting that he use condoms or use other low-risk behavior may result in violence, rejection, or abandonment. Counselors need to be clear with clients about the relative risk of transmission for different sexual activities by providing accurate, factual information about safer sex practices and low-risk behaviors. However, it is crucial to deal with issues of self-esteem and empowerment so that African-American women will feel that they can make and act on decisions that will be life-enhancing and self-protective. Because the identity of African-American women is so often based upon their relationship with others, the counselor may find support for behavior change by appealing to the woman's sense of responsibility to children and family.

The needs of African-American lesbians must also be addressed by the CMHC worker, in spite of the low incidence of HIV disease within this group. They, too, are faced with some risk of HIV infection. Therefore, it is incumbent upon counselors to become knowledgeable about issues related to sexual orientation and sexual behavior and to be able to discuss these comfortably and nonjudgmentally. It may be advisable for counselors to make referrals for services that are specifically designed for or run by gays and lesbians.

Using Cultural Strengths

Many cultural strengths exist within the African-American community which can be applied to clients dealing with HIV infection. Among these are spirituality, family and group interrelatedness, and values of competence and excellence. Many of these cultural strengths may have been "forgotten" in the midst of initially dealing with the crisis of HIV infection.

A CMHC clinician can help the client identify and use cultural strengths that exist in the African-American community. For example, many people with AIDS affirm that spirituality is instrumental in their coping with the disease. Although African-American churches have sometimes not been very supportive of people living with AIDS, an increasing number are becoming actively involved in providing care. Clients may wish to attend such a church. They may explore their spirituality on their own through reading, listening to inspirational music, and fellowship with other like-minded persons. Participation in support groups may help the client maintain positive behavior change and use effective coping mechanisms.

Strengthening ties with family members and friends and finding satisfying and enjoyable ways to be with them have also been identified as critical in coping with HIV disease. Clients can be encouraged to spend time with family and friends who can help them to maintain a positive attitude and sense of hope, and who can be accepting of times when the client is not at his or her best.

Promoting a positive self-image and building on pride in their cultural heritage may also enable clients to feel more connected to their community. Helping clients to identify the larger African-American community as a resource can further support their efforts to maintain and improve their health and deal with other relevant life issues.

The Need for Self-Assessment

African-American clients who have HIV disease or AIDS provide multiple challenges for counselors at CMHCs. It is important that, throughout the work, individual counselors, as well as the agency at large, engage in ongoing self-assessment to confront their attitudes about African-Americans, AIDS, substance abuse, homosexuality and bisexuality, racism, and families in poverty. The counselors' own cultural experiences will affect how they perceive the lives of their clients. Staff members must avoid the tendency to see the African-American client, who may be different because of cultural background, income level, education, HIV status, family situation, or sexual orientation, as inferior or less deserving than others. This attitude may be conveyed subtly, if not overtly, to the client and will interfere with the development of a therapeutic relationship.

It is important for CMHC clinicians to know specific techniques and approaches that have been found to be effective when working with African-American clients who are living with AIDS. However, it is equally important to understand and address the race, class, and gender issues at work in the environment which places African-American clients at risk for HIV disease. This provides an appropriate and informed context for development of effective, nonracist CMHC services.

Willingness on the part of the staff and the agency to gain cultural knowledge about themselves and African-Americans, to actively work for credibility in the African-American community, and to implement culturally sensitive and relevant programming will facilitate the development of a healthier African-American community that can more successfully battle the AIDS epidemic.

Latinos and HIV/AIDS

Working with Latino clients provides challenges for CMHC staff who are from a different racial or ethnic background and who may face language as well as cultural barriers when working with this population.

Transmission of HIV among Latinos

The incidence of AIDS among homosexual and bisexual males is two to three times higher in Latinos than among white men. Statistics on sexually transmitted diseases (STDs) suggest a persistence of high-risk behaviors among these Latino men. One study indicates that rates of rectal gonorrhea in homosexual/bisexual Latino men have not shown the decline seen among white homosexuals/bisexuals attending STD clinics in New York and San Francisco. Injection drug use is one of the most significant routes of infection for Latinos.

Latina women account for 20 percent of all reported AIDS cases among women in the United States. Studies indicate a higher rate of HIV infection among Latinos living on the East coast and in Puerto Rico than elsewhere in the United States. A high percentage are injecting drug users or have partners who are injecting drug users.

Adolescents born to Puerto Rican families in the continental United States and acculturated to Anglo norms show the highest teen pregnancy rate among all Latinos in the United States and may be at greater risk of HIV infection than nonacculturated adolescents. Also, never-married Latina women are less likely than other Latina women and single Anglo women to use prevention measures. Finally, because many Mexican-American and Puerto Rican women are sterilized to prevent pregnancy, they may not see a need for barrier contraceptives.

Considerations and Strategies for Effective Interventions with Clients from the Latino Population

When initiating work with Latino clients in community mental health settings, standard intake procedures should be used in gathering data. Making assumptions on the basis of ethnicity is both inaccurate and inappropriate. However, there are critical areas that must be explored to gather a thorough psychosocial and developmental history so that accurate formulation and treatment planning can be done.

Key Cultural Considerations in Working with Latino Clients with HIV/AIDS

- Country of origin
- Language use and dominance
- Natural support systems
- Social network data
- Values and cultural norms

Country of Origin

With foreign-born Latinos, including those born in Puerto Rico, it is important to explore the client's migration history. In the case of Latinos born in the United States a similar migration history should be obtained regarding the client's family, including a determination of how many generations ago the move occurred. Furthermore, the counselor should explore the client's experiences in the United States related to discrimination or racism.

Language Use

Identification of a primary language is important in caring for Latino clients. When a Latino client, fluent in English, is seen by a monolingual Anglo community mental health worker, the existence of a mother tongue may be overlooked. When Latino clients are not fluent in English, staff may assume that the client speaks Spanish. Spanish is the primary language in most Latin American countries; the exceptions are Brazil, the Guyanas, Haiti, and other Caribbean nations. Indigenous languages abound in Mexico and Central and South America, while Yoruba and other African languages have influence in Puerto Rico, Cuba, the Dominican Republic, and other Caribbean countries.

Language congruence is important for the effective delivery of mental health services. Among the approaches that can be used to overcome language barriers, the most effective in descending order are: (1) providing the service with bilingual/bicultural staff; (2) using trained mental health interpreters (simultaneous or consecutive); and (3) teaching Spanish to the providers.

CMHC staff should determine whether clients are English-dominant, Spanish-dominant, or bilingual. Even for English-dominant clients, it is important to know which language was spoken at home and what type of schooling the client has had (bilingual or English-only programs). CMHC staff should be aware that Spanish-dominant or bilingual clients speaking English may invest much energy in correct expression, thus giving precedence to the cognitive aspect of communication over the affective component. Clients may then appear constricted or flat. Research has shown that Anglo therapists evaluating and treating such clients tend to overpathologize and misdiagnose them.

Clients may also use bilingualism as a defensive structure, using one language to communicate and reserving another as the emotional language. Clients may discuss emotionally difficult topics in their nondominant language as a way of maintaining some emotional distance. At other times, clients may use the dominant language to access special memories or experiences. Even if the clinician is monolingual, it may be useful to allow clients to think out loud in their dominant, emotional language to facilitate their access to, and organization of, meaningful material.

Natural Support Systems

The availability of natural support systems may be crucial in helping clients cope with an HIV diagnosis. An assessment of the social network should include a list of friends and acquaintances, indicating their ethnic background and, where appropriate, sexual orientation. In the case of Latino homosexual clients, it is important to determine which heterosexual friends are *entendidos,* that is, persons who know about and support their sexual orientation.

The current state of relationships with the family is particularly important. Both family meetings and genograms are useful assessment and therapeutic techniques that can be used. When it is not possible to interview the family because of geographic distance or rejection of the client, use of a genogram is recommended to gain an understanding of family dynamics and relations.

The CMHC worker should also establish whether the client has attributed family status to non-blood-related individuals, as this is frequently done in the Latino culture and, particularly so, by Latino homosexuals. If such is the case, then staff should treat these family members accordingly and include them in the assessment and therapeutic process.

A history of intimate relationships is important. If the client is currently in a relationship, the clinician should explore whether the partner is Latino or non-Latino. If the partner is non-Latino, the clinician should explore how the couple deals with their cultural differences and how these differences affect the couple's life style. How the client deals with racism, ethnocentrism, addictions, and homophobia may be seen in the client's interpersonal relations and choice of friends and partners. This will also influence the client's selection of a therapist when a choice is available.

Latino clients will likely be forced to choose between male/female, straight/gay, or the infrequently available Latino counselors. Some will give priority to ethnicity, while others will favor gender or sexual orientation. Still others may choose counselors with considerable substance abuse treatment experience, regardless of ethnic background. This forced choice should be explored in the assessment process, as it may illuminate therapeutic issues. When the selection results in a discordant therapeutic dyad, the therapist must be aware of, and sensitive to, the power differential that exists between himself or herself and the client.

Other Considerations

It is always important to consider specific values, attitudes, norms, and expectations in designing treatment plans. In planning interventions for Latino men who engage in homosexual sex, CMHC staff need to address the way individuals identify themselves as being gay, or bisexual, or just having sex with men. Many Latino males who have sexual relations with other men may reject or discount messages that imply that they are gay or homosexual.

CMHC clinicians should be aware that reliance on Euro-American relationship models where women are assertive and independent might be uncomfortable and culturally inappropriate for Latina women. Interventions should assist Latinos in translating knowledge and awareness of coping skills into effective behavioral repertoires. For some women, the emphasis may lie more with nonverbal than verbal skills. Possible negative impact on the family, especially on children, may increase the motivation of Latino men and women to accept treatment. Machismo may be useful among men because the cultural value emphasizes their role of responsibility for and protection of the family.

If possible, the CMHC staff should offer clients a choice of either English or Spanish counselors. If the counselor has limited command of Spanish, he or she should avoid literal translations. Monocultural/bilingual clinicians should avoid regionalisms in language and be aware of the educational level and socioeconomic status of clients, as it should influence their choice of words, images, and metaphors.

Review Questions

1. Name one feature of an intervention that would most distinguish a culturally competent provider from a culturally sensitive provider.

2. How might a client respond when confronted with a CMHC staff person who believes that all people should be treated alike?

3. Compare the incidence of AIDS among homosexual and bisexual Latino men to that among Anglo men.

References and Suggested Readings

Abad, V., Ramos, J., & Boyce, E. (1974). A model for the delivery of mental health services to Spanish-speaking minorities. *American Journal of Orthopsychiatry, 44,* 584–595.

Amaro, H. (1995). Love, sex and power: Considering women's realities in HIV prevention. *American Psychologist, 50*(6), 437–447.

Amaro, H., Montano-Lopez, R., & Pares-Avila, J.A. (1989). *Sexual and Contraceptive Knowledge, Attitudes, and Practices among Hispanics: Implications for AIDS Prevention.* Rockville, MD: National Institute on Drug Abuse.

Aoki, B.K. (1989). Cross cultural counseling: The extra dimension. In J.W. Dilley, C. Pies, & M. Helquist (Eds.), *Face to Face: A Guide to AIDS Counseling.* San Francisco: AIDS Health Project, University of California.

Boswell, J., Hexter, R., & Reinish, J. (Eds.) (in press). *Hispanic Culture: Implications for AIDS Prevention in Sexuality and Disease: Metaphors, Perceptions and Behavior in the AIDS Era.* New York: Oxford University Press.

Bowser, B.P., Fullilove, M.T., & Fullilove, R.E. (1990). African American youth and AIDS high risk behavior: The social context and barriers to prevention. *Youth and Society, 22,* 54–66.

Carballo-Dieguez, A. (1989). Hispanic culture, gay male culture, and AIDS: Counseling implications. *Journal of Counseling and Development, 68*(2), 26–30.

Carballo-Dieguez, A., & Dolezal, C. (1994). Contrasting types of Puerto Rican men who have sex with men (MSM). *Journal of Psychology and Human Sexuality, 6*(4), 41–67.

Carrier, J.M., & Magaña, J.R. (1991). Use of ethnosexual data on men of Mexican origin for HIV/AIDS prevention programs. *The Journal of Sex Research, 28,* 189–202.

Ceballos-Capitaine, A., Szapocznik, J., Blaney, N.T., Morgan, R.O., Millon, C., & Eisdorfer, C. (1990). Ethnicity, emotional distress, stress-related disruption, and coping among HIV seropositive gay males. *Hispanic Journal of Behavioral Sciences, 12,* 135–152.

Centers for Disease Control and Prevention. (1997). *HIV/AIDS Surveillance Report. 8*(2).

Comas-Diaz, L. (1985). Culturally relevant issues and treatment implications for Hispanics. In D.R. Koslow & E. Salett (Eds.), *Crossing Cultures in Mental Health.* (31–48). Washington, D.C.: SIETAR International.

Duh, S. (1991). *Blacks and AIDS: Causes and Origins.* Newbury Park, CA: Sage Publications.

Espin, O.M. (1984). Cultural and historical influences on sexuality in Hispanic/Latin women: Implications for psychotherapy. In C. Vance (Ed.), *Towards a New Politics of Sexuality.* London: Routledge & P. Kegan.

Gordon, S.M. (1995). Hispanic cultural health beliefs and folk remedies, *Journal of Holistic Nursing, 12*(3), 307–322.

Hahn, R.A., & Castro, K.G. (1989). The health care status of Latino populations in the U.S.: A brief review. In O. Martinez-Maza, D.M. Shin, & H. Banks (Eds.), *Latinos and AIDS: A National Strategy Symposium.* (1–7). Los Angeles: University of California.

Jones, R.L. (1991). *Black Psychology* (3rd ed.). CA Berkeley: Cobb and Henry.

Jue, S. (1987). Identifying and meeting the needs of minority clients with AIDS. In C.G. Leukefeld & M. Fimbres (Eds.), *Responding to AIDS.* Silver Spring, MD: National Association of Social Workers.

Kalichman, S.C., Rompa, D., & Coley, B. (1996). Experimental component analysis of a behavioral HIV/AIDS prevention intervention for inner-city women. *Journal of Consulting and Clinical Psychology, 64*(4), 687–693.

McBride, D. (1991). *From TB to AIDS.* New York: State University Press.

Parés-Avila, J.A., & Montano-López, R. (1994). Issues in the psychosocial care of Latino gay men with HIV infection. In S.A. Cadwell, R.A. Burnham, & M. Forstein (Eds.), *Therapists on the Front Line: Psychotherapy with Gay Men in the Age of AIDS.* (339–377). Washington, D.C.: American Psychiatric Press.

Pearlberg, G. (1991). *Women, AIDS, and Communities: A Guide for Action.* Metuchen, NJ: Women's Action Alliance and Scarecrow Press.

Phillips, F.K. (1990). NTU psychotherapy: An Afrocentric approach. *The Journal of Black Psychotherapy, 17*(1), 55–74.

Quimby, E. (1993). Obstacles to reducing AIDS among African Americans. *Journal of Black Psychology, 19*(2), 215–222.

Selik, R.M., Castro, K.G., Pappaioanou, M., & Buehler, J.W. (1989). Birthplace and the risk of AIDS among Hispanics in the United States. *American Journal of Public Health, 77,* 69–72.

Schneider, B.E., & Stoller, N.E. (1995). *Women Resisting AIDS.* Philadelphia: Temple University Press.

Stevenson, G.C. (1994). The psychology of sexual racism and AIDS: An ongoing saga of distrust and the "sexual other." *Journal of Black Studies, 25*(1), 62–80.

Tolliver, D., & Kupona Network Women's Coalition (1992). *Sister Rap: A Safer Sex Curriculum for African-American Women Using the Q-Sort Pictographic Method of Evaluation: A Technical Manual.* Unpublished manuscript.

Walters, J.L., Canady, R., & Stein, T. (1994). Evaluating multicultural approaches in HIV/AIDS educational material. *AIDS Education and Prevention, 6*(5), 446–453.

Weeks, M.R., Schensul, J.J., Williams, S.S., Singer, M., & Grier, M. (1995). AIDS prevention for African-American and Latina women: Building culturally and gender-appropriate intervention. *AIDS Education and Prevention. 7*(3), 251–263.

Chapter 17

Treating Persons with Serious and Persistent Mental Illness

Martha A. Friedrich, Ph.D., and
John A. Grannan, M.A.

Overview

This chapter examines why mental illness is a risk factor for HIV infection and why and how to do a risk assessment of all clients. Also presented are issues to consider when treating HIV-infected clients, including how both clients and staff are affected and the impact of having an HIV-positive client on an inpatient unit. There is discussion on ways that HIV can affect pharmacological interventions with clients, focusing on problems with side effects and proper dosage. HIV educational interventions for persons with mental illness are also described.

Learning Objectives

1. To specify at least three reasons why mental illness is a risk factor for HIV infection.

2. To list the areas that should be covered in doing an HIV risk-factor assessment.

3. To describe at least three essential elements of HIV education for persons with serious and persistent mental illness.

Outline

I. Diagnostic Issues

    A. Why mental illness is a risk factor for infection

    B. The need for an HIV risk assessment

    C. Neurological symptoms causing misdiagnosis

    D. Emergence of AIDS phobia and AIDS panic

II. Therapeutic Issues

    A. Dealing with life-threatening illness

    B. Special problems on CMHC units

        1. Limited participation

        2. Limit-setting and minimizing new stimuli

        3. Need to modify visitation policies

        4. Supervised living arrangements

        5. Protecting client confidentiality

        6. Use of universal precautions

III. Pharmacological Issues

    A. Lower dosages

    B. Choosing medications

IV. HIV Educational Needs of Persons with Mental Illness

    A. Teaching risk reduction

        1. Assertiveness training

        2. Negotiating safer sex

        3. Distribution and proper use of condoms

        4. Considering cultural background

        5. Gender-separate education groups

    B. Responding to fears and concerns of clients

Diagnostic Issues

Why Mental Illness Is a Risk Factor for Infection

Many persistently and severely mentally ill persons may be at high-risk for HIV infection. Research studies have found that HIV seroprevalence among psychiatric inpatients is higher than in the general population. Several characteristics of inpatients may contribute to this. Cognitive impairment, poor judgment, affective instability, and impulsivity are likely to result in behavior that includes unsafe sexual practices and various forms of substance abuse. The passivity often seen in persons with chronic mental illness can leave them vulnerable to exploitation by others. Persons from disadvantaged social and economic backgrounds may be more susceptible to sexual coercion and abuse.

Factors That May Increase Risk for HIV Infection

- Cognitive impairment
- Poor judgment
- Affective instability
- Impulsivity
- Passivity
- Disadvantaged social and economic status
- Increased substance abuse
- Interaction with other individuals with high risk behaviors

Persons with mental illness living in low-income, inner-city areas are at high risk for HIV infection. Individuals living in these locations are likely to be exposed to injection drugs and crack cocaine. Sharing needles and syringes are not the only ways for a substance abuser to become infected. Impaired judgment from the effects of drugs, including alcohol, can put a person at greater sexual risk. Adolescents hospitalized for psychiatric reasons may have a high risk for HIV infection because of increased substance abuse and sexual activity.

Persons with mental illness also are more prone to interact with other populations with high-risk behavior for HIV in various psychiatric facilities, homeless shelters, jails, and forensic units. Research shows that state psychiatric facilities will likely have a higher incidence of HIV-infected clients who have pre-existing schizophrenia and bipolar disorders. Persons incarcerated in state and county prisons also have a much higher prevalence of HIV infection than that found in the general population.

The Need for an HIV Risk Assessment

Given that mental illness can increase the risk of infection, clients should be carefully assessed. An assessment of HIV risk factors should be completed as part of the history taking at a community mental health center (CMHC), whether it be for inpatient or outpatient treatment. This assessment process can be beneficial for the client and for treatment planning. While the staff person learns relevant information about the client's life-style, the client may gain insight about his or her own risk factors.

HIV Risk Assessment for Persons with Mental Illness

- HIV awareness
- Substance use history
- Sexual/physical abuse
- Sexual history:
    - Frequency
    - Number of partners
    - Gender of partners
    - Risk behaviors of partners
    - Kind of sexual activity
    - Exchanging sex for drugs or money
    - History of sexually transmitted diseases
    - Use of condoms

An assessment can be done by asking a series of questions to determine possible risk behaviors. The first questions determine the client's knowledge about HIV/AIDS, focusing on transmission and any behavioral changes he or she may have made as a result of that information. Adult clients should be asked if they have been tested for the HIV antibody and if they want to be tested. They should also be asked if they would like to be tested now and if they can specify the reasons why they do or do not choose testing. The responses to these questions may give a clinician additional knowledge about the client's judgment and level of awareness.

Some clients may not be able to give reliable information at the time of the history taking because of thought disorders, paranoia, hallucinations, and poor memory. In these cases, it would be better to wait to complete a risk assessment until after the presenting symptoms have been treated. Some clients may be reluctant to share such personal information about themselves with a stranger. It can be threatening for a client to admit to controversial and illegal (in some states) behavior, such as homosexual activity and illicit use of drugs. Several interviews may be required to establish enough rapport to elicit the information.

The following questions are general screening questions for major risk factors.

HIV Risk Assessment Questions

- Can you tell me how the virus that causes AIDS is transmitted?
- Are you worried about getting AIDS? If yes, why?
- Have you ever been tested for the virus that causes AIDS? If yes, when?
- What were the test results?
- Do you want to be tested now? Why or why not?
- Did you have a blood transfusion before 1986?
- Have you ever injected drugs? If yes, when?
- How much alcohol do you consume on a weekly basis?
- Do you use any other drugs now or have you in the past?
- Have you ever been physically or sexually abused or raped?
- Have you ever had sex? (If no, end the assessment.)
- How often have you had sex during the past year?
- How many different sexual partners have you had in the past five years?
- Were they men, women, or both?
- Have you ever had sex with someone who injected drugs or had multiple sexual partners or other high-risk behavior for AIDS?
- Have you ever exchanged sex for money or drugs?
- Have you ever had a sexually transmitted disease?
- Can you tell me how to use condoms properly?
- Have you ever used condoms? If yes, how often? If no, why not?

A thorough substance use history also needs to be done, one in which use of all possible substances is covered. (See Chapter 18, "Treating Persons Who Use Drugs.") Even if the client reports being in recovery from either alcohol or other drugs, the risk associated with past behavior needs to be recognized. This would also be an opportunity to determine if any sexual partners were substance users. Many women have been infected by sexual partners who were either former or current users.

A risk assessment should address sexual and physical abuse, in both childhood and adulthood. Rape should be mentioned specifically because some people may not perceive this to be sexual abuse. Like other survivors of childhood abuse, persons who are also mentally ill will probably have low self-esteem and a sense of powerlessness over their sexuality. They are vulnerable to sexual exploitation by others and some may act out with aggressive and compulsive sexual activities. If the client says that this has occurred, this would, of course, be a therapeutic issue to be dealt with outside of the context of this assessment.

An assessment should include questions to determine the frequency of sexual contacts and the number, gender, and risk behavior of the partners. The kind of sexual activity needs to be considered since intercourse, both vaginal and anal, is riskier than oral sex or mutual masturbation. A history of buying or selling sex would increase the likelihood of HIV infection. The client should also be asked about any history of sexually transmitted diseases (STDs) since research shows a correlation between STDs and increased risk for HIV infection. A complete sexual history should include the client's knowledge about, and use of, condoms.

Neurological Symptoms Can Cause Misdiagnosis

Problems in Diagnosing

- HIV can mimic diverse syndromes.
- HIV can be misdiagnosed.
- Rule out opportunistic infections.
- Medications can cause symptoms.
- Do not rely on early neuropsychological signs.
- An antibody test may be needed.

Be aware that the neurological symptoms you may attribute to mental illness may be caused by HIV infection. (See Chapter 9, "Neuropsychological Functioning in HIV Disease.") HIV infection of the brain has the ability to mimic diverse syndromes and may cause some difficulty in making a proper diagnosis. Because it can affect the central nervous system early in the course of infection, HIV may cause problems in thinking and memory. Other cases of an HIV-related delirium or dementia may present with mainly psychotic symptoms, including delusions and hallucinations. If the presence of HIV infection is not known, these clients may be incorrectly diagnosed. This is even more likely to happen in a person with a history of mental illness. Psychotic symptoms may be assumed to reflect the mental illness when in fact they are the manifestation of HIV disease.

Opportunistic infections that can affect the brain of an HIV-infected person, such as toxoplasmosis, cryptococcosis, or a primary brain lymphoma, can cause psychotic reactions and affect memory, vision, coordination, and speech patterns. These infections, if misdiagnosed and left untreated, can result in death. Some medications often prescribed for HIV, such as AZT, Bactrim/Septra, or Zovirax can cause anxiety, depression, confusion, or insomnia and should be considered in an evaluation by a physician. The early neuropsychological signs (cognitive, motor, and behavioral) of HIV infection can be confused with common presenting symptoms of mental illness. Some early physical symptoms of HIV such as weight loss, shortness of breath, night sweats, oral infections, and changes in skin conditions should indicate the need for further evaluation. Clients who report high-risk behavior or have lived in areas reporting high incidence of HIV should be referred for antibody testing.

If the client does not report a previous positive test for the HIV antibody, then a test may be needed to rule it out. Most states will require the client's permission before a test can be given. There are some states that allow testing without an individual's permission in certain circumstances, usually when the person is incarcerated or under psychiatric care. All facilities and private healthcare providers should be aware of the law in their respective states.

Emergence of AIDS Phobia and AIDS Panic

AIDS Phobia or AIDS Panic

- Fears about AIDS can cause delusions.
- Delusions can result from guilt.
- Obsessional or paranoid history is a higher risk.
- Obsessive-compulsive disorder may develop.
- There may be conflict with sexual orientation.
- Reports of factitious AIDS may develop.
- AIDS may be considered a conspiracy.
- Use antibody tests to rule out HIV.
- Underlying mental illness must be treated.

An issue to be aware of is the emergence of AIDS panic among persons who are mentally ill. Delusions presented by persons with mental dysfunction can be a combination of psychopathology and current events. As AIDS becomes a fixture in the public consciousness, it may be increasingly incorporated into the delusional material of persons who are mentally ill. Clients without evidence of compromised immune status and without a history of high-risk behavior may present with a complaint of having AIDS. With the stigma associated with having AIDS, the delusion of having AIDS may help someone whose sense of guilt about past behavior needs a tangible form.

Clients with a history of premorbid obsessional and paranoid personality features may be at higher risk for developing what is being called an AIDS phobia or AIDS panic. Other individuals may develop an obsessive-compulsive disorder in which concern about AIDS played a central role. Men with a history of homosexual activity may experience panic. In such cases, psychotherapeutic intervention should consider any conflict with sexual orientation.

Cases of factitious AIDS have also been reported and may represent an attempt by an individual to deny a psychological decompensation by expressing it as a physical disorder. There have been reported incidents of clients refuting the existence of AIDS, believing it to be a conspiracy by the government and doctors to discourage people from having sex or possibly just a scheme for condom companies to get rich.

For those clients who are delusional or obsessional, providing an HIV antibody test is appropriate. Family members may be relieved at the negative test result, but the client is usually not convinced by that information. Successful treatment of underlying disorders is usually the most effective way to eliminate the delusion and reduce the anxiety.

Therapeutic Issues

Dealing with Life-Threatening Illness

Therapeutic Issues of Life-Threatening Illness

- Staff discomfort
- Issues of debilitating illness
- Increase of suicide risk
- Referral to HIV support groups
- Client interaction with HIV physician

Many CMHC workers may not be used to dealing with life-threatening illness, and surveys show that they are often uncomfortable. Some health professionals may have chosen to work in mental health to avoid dealing with the terminally ill. In addition, some of the staff may have difficulty dealing with the increased dependency associated with debilitating disease when the usual goal of mental health treatment is increased independence of clients. These issues are, of course, also psychologically challenging to the clients themselves.

Terminal illness has long been understood to increase the risk of suicidal behavior. This is perhaps even more true with HIV, its associated stigma, and loss of supports. (See Chapter 13, "Suicide Assessment and Intervention with Persons Infected with HIV.") It is not known how this risk relates to the suicide risk associated with some mental illness, but it is reasonable to assume that the combined risk is greater than either alone.

Clients may benefit from efforts to enhance social support when isolated. Although many existing HIV support groups may resist the possible disruption of including persons with mental illness, these groups can be a valuable opportunity for clients to share knowledge and feelings about HIV infection with others. Many times, a person with a history of mental illness will find it difficult to assimilate into an existing support group for persons with HIV/AIDS. Most of the other group members will not have been treated for a mental illness and may feel uncomfortable including a person who has in their group. The HIV support group members may not view the person with mental illness as a peer and will probably be overly critical or suspicious about information shared by him or her. Experience has shown that they will also not be included in socializing outside the group because of their perceived difference and concern about their behavior. If possible, specialized groups should be developed by the CMHC for this unique population.

Many of the psychological challenges associated with HIV disease arise from the uncertainty and unpredictability of its course. Client passivity or physician discomfort with mental illness may prevent the necessary exchange of information between these two individuals to alleviate some of this uncertainty. It may then fall to CMHC workers to communicate this important information in the context of a "safe" relationship where the individual feels comfortable asking questions and expressing emotional responses.

Special Problems on CMHC Units

Considerations

- Participation may be limited.
- Activities should not put the client at risk.
- Limit setting and behavior modification may be needed.

- New routine should minimize new stimuli.
- Visitation policies may need to be modified.
- Family and friends may need additional support.
- Where to discharge may be in question.
- Keeping HIV status secret is stressful.
- Client's confidentiality must be protected.
- Universal precautions must be used for all clients.
- Clients should be told of universal precaution policy.

HIV infection poses special problems for people being treated in community mental health facilities. Fatigue and confusion experienced by HIV-infected clients may limit their participation in group activities. Personal involvement in unit activities by such clients will depend upon their cognitive and physical abilities. Cooking instruction and pet-assisted therapy may have to be modified to protect immune-compromised clients from exposure to pathogens, such as *Salmonella* (from raw chicken or turkey), *Cryptosporidium* (from raw vegetables), and *Toxoplasma gondii* (transmitted by cats).

Clients with dementia may be unable to respond to limit setting used to promote behavioral change. Decreased memory, increased impulsiveness, and perseveration may reduce the effectiveness of behavior modification. Nevertheless, these clients may be helped by establishing routines that minimize new stimuli. Those clients who are physically healthy and exhibiting symptoms of depression need to be encouraged to actively participate in unit activities. Those with advanced debility and dementia should not be expected to be as active as other clients and should be allowed to withdraw when needed.

Visitation policies for CMHC inpatient programs may have to be modified to allow more time with family and friends as time becomes more precious. Families and significant others are often struggling with their grief along with issues of sexuality and life-styles. Family members should be encouraged to seek referrals for their own mental health treatment and to any appropriate support groups.

Many clients with HIV/AIDS will need some type of supervised living arrangements after treatment in an inpatient program. Problems with discharge because of limited community resources may cause clients to stay at the facility beyond the point of documented need.

Inpatients may have problems interacting with others if they do not disclose their status and feel inhibited by the burden of their secret. If they disclose their status, others, particularly those with paranoid symptoms, may cause interpersonal problems on the unit. In any case, it is imperative that staff respect client confidentiality about the HIV diagnosis and not disclose to anyone who does not need to know it to provide treatment.

Criteria for implementing seclusion and restraint procedures should not be modified for those who are known to be HIV-infected. Universal precautions should be part of the seclusion and restraint procedures when any client is assaultive. Clients with HIV must not think that their behavior will have different consequences than that of other noninfected clients because of staff fear of infection. All clients should be told in advance, perhaps at an orientation, that staff will use universal precautions such as gloves and any other required protective gear as needed. It should be emphasized that these precautions will be used in incidents concerning all clients. Staff members should be vigilant to protect the confidentiality of an HIV-infected client and not do or say anything to compromise a client's right to privacy.

Pharmacological Issues

Pharmacological Issues for Clients with HIV/AIDS

- Lower dosage is recommended.
- Avoid drugs with high anticholinergic side effects.
- Methylphenidate (Ritalin) is useful for depression and dementia.
- Benzodiazepines and neuroleptics may worsen dementia.
- Drug interactions should be considered.

Drug tolerance in HIV-infected individuals is reduced, so most psychoactive drugs should be given in lower dosages than given with the general population of psychiatric clients. Most recommendations suggest roughly half of the adult dose. Drugs with anticholinergic side effects, such as dry mouth and difficulty with urination, should be avoided. There are antidepressants with few or no anticholinergic side effects, such as the tricyclic drug Norpramin (desipramine) and other types of antidepressants such as Prozac (fluoxetine), Desyrel (trazodone), and Wellbutrin (bupropion). Although Prozac can cause side effects of insomnia and appetite suppression, which could already be a problem for someone with HIV, it can stimulate those with apathy or lethargy. People with a history of liver damage, including hepatitis, should not take Prozac. Desyrel is extremely sedating and also may cause unwanted painful erections in males. Wellbutrin should be used with caution because of the increased risk of seizures in persons with HIV who are affected by central nervous system illnesses.

In persons with either HIV-related dementia or depression, Ritalin (methylphenidate) has been used with good results, especially in those with cognitive and motor slowing. Possible side effects of Ritalin include insomnia, appetite suppression, and tremors.

Benzodiazepines, such as Valium (diazepam) and Xanax (alprazolam), may worsen memory problems in clients with dementia. There have also been reports of adverse reactions to the benzodiazepine drug Ativan (lorazepam) in persons with dementia, resulting in hallucinations and severe cognitive difficulties. Antipsychotic drugs, such as Thorazine (chlorpromazine) and Haldol (haloperidol), have been used with success in most cases, but some persons with dementia can be susceptible to side effects and toxicity.

In addition to concerns about side effects, the possibilities of drug interactions should also be considered. People with HIV infection are likely to be taking multiple medications including reverse transcriptase inhibitors and/or protease inhibitors as well as treatment and/or prophylaxis for opportunistic illnesses. These drugs may interact with each other or with psychotropic medications. Up-to-date comprehensive drug reference guides (e.g., Bartlett, 1996), which include drug interaction warnings, should be available to mental health center staff. A comprehensive list of an individual's current medications should be obtained before prescribing additional drugs.

HIV Educational Needs of Persons with Mental Illness

Educational Interventions

- Cognitive and emotional deficits may impair learning.
- Increase in knowledge does not guarantee behavior change.
- Education should focus on risk reduction.
- Assertiveness training should be an integral part of education.
- Challenges of negotiating safer sex should be confronted.
- Information about condoms and their availability must be provided.
- Cultural background must be considered.
- Separate groups for men and women should be established.

People with major mental illnesses can and should learn about HIV. However, the cognitive or emotional deficits of these persons may impair their ability to understand and use information about AIDS. Even when they admit to high-risk behaviors, they also frequently report a low level of fear of contracting HIV. Therefore, standard community education efforts may be inadequate. The special educational needs of persons with a severe mental illness may best be served at mental health treatment facilities.

Teaching Risk Reduction

An increase in AIDS knowledge does not guarantee changes in behavior or the cessation of activities that can spread HIV. People who know that they are infected may think that it is no longer necessary to worry about protecting themselves. Some people have reported that they do not care if they infect others; they continue to have unprotected sex. These individuals need to know that their own health may suffer if they receive an additional exposure to HIV. Their health is also threatened by infection from other STDs.

Those teaching risk reduction to persons with mental illness need to take some factors into consideration. For those with a history of previous sexual abuse, their sexual behavior may be a preferred means of socializing and attracting the attention of others. Encouraging such individuals to limit their sexual activity and to use condoms may be asking too much. They may fear that losing their sexual partners will mean losing intimacy or attention. Some may also think of sex as a source of immediate pleasure, and a recommendation of abstinence or monogamy may seem impossible. Someone with low self-esteem and depressive tendencies may also refuse to practice safer sex in what could be viewed as a passive suicidal gesture.

Risk reduction must include the teaching of assertive behaviors. Persons with mental illness often demonstrate passive-aggressive behaviors. Some may have previously attended assertiveness training groups and would benefit from a refresher course. Negotiating safer sex with a partner requires assertive behaviors. Role-playing is an effective way to improve a client's assertiveness and self-esteem.

Information about the proper use of condoms must be taught to clients. Some persons with mental illness may also have problems with manual dexterity caused by the side effects of their medications. Other clients may have impaired intellectual functioning. Any training about condoms must take into consideration the individual capabilities of each client.

Distribution of free or low-cost condoms is also important. Many clients will not have the money to buy condoms or access to purchase them. As in the general population, some will also find it difficult to buy condoms in public because it could be embarrassing. Assertiveness role-playing can help clients to overcome their anxiety.

Another variable to consider is the cultural background of each client. Studies are showing that persons from varying ethnic backgrounds will respond differently to education about risk reduction. For many women, especially those from Hispanic families, negotiating or even requesting safer sex can be difficult. Low self-esteem and a cultural bias against women's sexuality can make it extremely challenging for a female with a mental illness to be assertive with her sexual partner.

If possible, sex education, specifically training about HIV/AIDS and safer sex, should be conducted in gender-segregated groups. The presence of men seems to intimidate some women, reducing their participation in groups and their learning. Gender-separate groups are particularly indicated in mental health facilities since persons with mental illnesses tend to be more conservative about sex roles in particular and sexuality in general.

Responding to Fears and Concerns of Clients

Dealing with Fears and Concerns

- Fear of contagion is normal.
- Transmission information should be disseminated.
- Paranoia may increase fears and concerns.
- Concerns are used as avoidance behavior.
- Staff should provide rumor control.
- Issues should be discussed in a group setting.
- Fears and concerns should not be ignored.
- All clients will suffer if issues are not addressed.

Many staff and clients will have concerns about being in contact with a person who is HIV-positive. Fear of contagion is a normal human reaction. Care must be taken to ensure that all clients are given information, both verbal and written, about the transmission of HIV/AIDS, emphasizing how the virus can and cannot be transmitted. Those clients with paranoid disorders would understandably be affected by the presence of an HIV-infected individual. Some clients may use their concerns as a way to avoid dealing with their own treatment-related issues.

To prevent AIDS from becoming a main issue on the unit, staff members need to provide "rumor control." A most effective way to deal with these fears and concerns, both rational and irrational, is in a group setting. The group can be focused on health issues, including sexuality, STDs, and HIV, or it can be in a client-staff

community meeting. It is important to talk about the fears and concerns and not
ignore them or pretend they are not present. These issues will not go away and, if
not dealt with by staff in a timely and sensitive manner, could have a detrimental
effect on the HIV-infected client as well as other clients.

Review Questions

1. Why may it be difficult to properly diagnose someone with HIV infection
who also has a psychiatric history and what should be done to prevent a possible
misdiagnosis?

2. Since having a client with HIV infection on an inpatient unit can affect
both staff and clients, what are some of the potential problems and what steps can
be taken to respond to them?

3. What are the essential elements of an HIV risk-reduction education program for clients with mental health illness and what issues need to be considered in
designing such a program?

References and Suggested Readings

Aruffo, J.F., Coverdale, J.H., Chacko, R.C., & Dworkin, R.J. (1990). Knowledge about AIDS
among women psychiatric outpatients. *Hospital and Community Psychiatry, 41,* 326–328.
Baer, J.W., Dwyer, P.C., & Lewitter-Koehler, S. (1988). Knowledge about AIDS among psychi-
atric inpatients. *Hospital and Community Psychiatry, 39,* 986–988.
Baer, J.W., Hall, J.M., Holm, K., & Lewitter-Koehler, S. (1987). Challenges in developing an
inpatient psychiatric program for patients with AIDS and ARC. *Hospital and Community
Psychiatry, 38,* 1299–1303.
Bartlett, J.G. (1996). *Pocket Book of Infectious Disease Therapy.* Baltimore: Williams & Wilkins.
Carmen, E., & Brady, S. (1990). AIDS risk and prevention for the chronic mentally ill. *Hospital
and Community Psychiatry, 41,* 652–657.
Cook, J.A., Razzano, L., Jayaraj, A., Myers, M., Nathanson, F., Stott, M.A., & Stein, M. (1994).
HIV-risk assessment for psychiatric rehabilitation clientele: Implications for community-
based services. *Psychosocial Rehabilitation Journal, 17*(4), 105–115.
Cournos, F., McKinnon, K., Meyer-Bahlburg, H., Guido, J., & Meyer, I. (1993). HIV risk activ-
ity among persons with severe mental illness: Preliminary findings. *Hospital and
Community Psychiatry, 44*(11), 1104–1106.
Cummings, M.A., Cummings, K.L., Rapaport, M.H., Atkinson, J.H., & Grant, I. (1987).
Acquired immunodeficiency syndrome presenting as schizophrenia. *The Western Journal of
Medicine, 146,* 615–618.
Empfield, M., Cournos, F., Meyer, I., McKinnon, K., Horwath, E., Silver, M., Schrage, H., &
Herman, R. (1993). HIV seroprevalence among homeless patients admitted to a psychiatric
inpatient unit. *American Journal of Psychiatry, 150*(1), 47–52.

Goisman, R.M., Kent, A.B., Montgomery, E.C., Cheevers, M.M., & Goldfinger, S.M. (1991). AIDS education for patients with chronic mental illness. *Community Mental Health Journal, 27,* 189–197.

Hanson, M., Kramer, T.H., Gross, W., Quintana, J., Li, P.W., & Asher, R. (1992). AIDS awareness and risk behaviors among dually disordered adults. *AIDS Education and Prevention, 4*(1), 41–51.

Horwath, E., Kramer, M., Cournos, F., Empfield, M., & Gewirtz, G. (1989). Clinical presentations of AIDS and HIV infection in state psychiatric facilities. *Hospital and Community Psychiatry, 40,* 502–506.

Kalichman, S.C., Kelly, J.A., Johnson, J.R., & Bulto, M. (1994). Factors associated with risk for HIV infection among chronic mentally ill adults. *American Journal of Psychiatry, 151*(2), 221–227.

Kalichman, S.C., Sikkema, K.J., Kelly, J.A., & Bulto, M. (1995). Use of a brief behavioral skills intervention to prevent HIV infection among chronic mentally ill adults. *Psychiatric Services, 46*(3), 275–280.

Katz, R.C., Watts, C., & Santman, J. (1994). AIDS knowledge and high risk behaviors in the chronic mentally ill. *Community Mental Health Journal, 30*(4), 395–402.

Kelly, J.A., Murphy, D.A., Bahr, G.R., Brasfield, T.L., Davis, D.R., Hauth, A.C., Morgan, M.G., Stevenson, L.Y., & Eilers, M.K. (1992). AIDS/HIV Risk Behavior among the Chronic Mentally Ill. *American Journal of Psychiatry, 149*(7), 886–889.

Knox, M.D., Boaz, T.L., Friedrich, M.A., & Dow, M.G. (1994). HIV risk factors for persons with serious mental illness. *Community Mental Health Journal, 30,* 551–563.

Mahorney, S.L., & Cavenar, J.O. (1988). A new and timely delusion: The complaint of having AIDS. *American Journal of Psychiatry, 145,* 1130–1132.

McKinnon, K., Cournos, F., Meyer-Bahlburg, H., Guido, H., Caraballo, L., Margoshes, E., Herman, R., Gruen, R., & Exner, T. (1993). Reliability of sexual risk interviews with psychiatric patients. *American Journal of Psychiatry, 150*(6), 972–974.

Rector, N.A., & Seeman, M.V. (1992). Schizophrenia and AIDS [Letter to the editor]. *Hospital and Community Psychiatry, 43*(2), 181.

Sacks, M.H., Perry, S., Graver, R., Shindledecker, R., & Hall, S. (1990). Self-reported HIV-related risk behaviors in acute psychiatric inpatients: A pilot study. *Hospital and Community Psychiatry, 41,* 1253–1255.

Seeman, M.V., Lang, M., & Rector, N. (1990). Chronic schizophrenia: A risk factor for HIV? *Canadian Journal of Psychiatry, 35,* 765–768.

Volavka, J., Convit, A., O'Donnell, J., Douyon, R., Evangelista, C., & Czobor, P. (1992). Assessment of risk behaviors for HIV infection among psychiatric patients. *Hospital and Community Psychiatry, 43,* 482–485.

Yudofsky, S., Hales, R., & Ferguson, T. (1991). *What You Need to Know about Psychiatric Drugs.* New York: Grove Weidenfeld.

Chapter 18

Treating Persons Who Use Drugs

Mark G. Winiarski, Ph.D.

Overview

This chapter is intended to familiarize community mental health center (CMHC) clinicians with treatment issues that arise when clients who use drugs are also HIV-positive. After a brief review of explanatory models of substance abuse and addiction, the focus is the relationship between substance abuse and HIV. Also included is information on assessment, treatment, and the impact of socioeconomic and cultural issues. The counselors' attitudes and abilities, the structure of the clinical setting, and the client's individual needs are all shown to be part of an effective therapeutic relationship.

Learning Objectives

1. To understand that the counselor's attitudes regarding a client's symptoms play an important role in the success of treating a substance user.

2. To show familiarity with various explanatory models for substance use.

3. To list two ways in which substance abuse is a risk behavior for HIV infection.

4. To demonstrate cultural sensitivity and open-mindedness to the experience of the HIV-positive substance user.

Outline

   I. Models of Substance Use and Addiction
     A. Biopsychosocial model
     B. Cognitive-behavioral model
     C. Medical model
     D. Psychodynamic model
     E. Integrated treatment

  II. Relationships Between Substance Abuse and HIV
     A. Exchange of body fluids via injecting drugs
     B. Disinhibiting effects of drugs
     C. Sex for drugs and drug money
     D. Sexual transmission from injecting drug user (IDU) to partners

 III. Socioeconomic and Cultural Issues
     A. Screening for substance use regardless of socioeconomic factors
     B. Sensitivity to cultural and subcultural norms

 IV. Assessment of HIV-Positive Clients with Histories of Substance Use
     A. Medical history
     B. Client's knowledge and compliance
     C. Cognitive functioning
     D. Psychiatric/psychological history
     E. History of substance use
     F. Psychosocial/cultural background and support systems

  V. Treatment Issues
     A. Integration of mental health and substance abuse treatments
     B. Case management issues
     C. Use of a flexible therapeutic framework

Models of Substance Use and Addiction

There are many different views regarding substance use. The following models are helpful in understanding why some people abuse drugs.

Models of Substance Abuse

- Biopsychosocial
- Cognitive-behavioral
- Medical
- Psychodynamic

Biopsychosocial Model

The most comprehensive way to understand substance use and addiction is the biopsychosocial model. In this model, substance abuse is a biopsychosocial condition, with biological and medical components as well as psychological, social, and community components. It is not sufficient to view the biological, psychological, and social aspects as three separate components because these elements interact. Given our current knowledge, we cannot say that a behavior is strictly biological or strictly psychological. For instance, studies indicate some persons may be genetically predisposed to alcoholism. But substance use behavior is determined by psychological and social factors as well. Researchers have noted that alcohol and drug use have many contributing factors (Institute of Medicine, 1990).

Understanding substance use in a biopsychosocial model is important because substance abuse treatment is moving toward integrated models that take all aspects of a client's functioning into account. Practitioners now believe a comprehensive program is needed for adequate treatment. For example, a client may be treated with drugs for an underlying psychiatric condition, with individual therapy that includes a cognitive-behavioral approach to relapse prevention, and with family therapy for interpersonal and social problems. Twelve-step programs are also often part of the treatment.

Cognitive-Behavioral Model

Many mental health counselors have training in a cognitive-behavioral model of substance abuse treatment. This model focuses on identifying distorted or erroneous thinking and the attitudes that derive from such thoughts that lead to inappropriate behavior. A person may act or think "automatically." In terms of drug use, a person may believe that, by using drugs, he or she will become more accepted by his or her peers. Or a person may believe that using drugs helps to improve coping. An excellent introduction to cognitive-behavioral techniques in work with persons with substance use problems is Miller and Rollnick's (1991) compilation of motivational approaches.

Another useful cognitive-behavioral treatment of substance use is relapse prevention, pioneered by Marlatt and Gordon (1985) and now adapted by many others. Treatment focuses on training recovering drug and alcohol users to recognize cognitive and situational cues that signal when they are in high-risk situations so that they may begin using positive coping techniques and make the choice not to use again.

Medical Model

Many of us have been taught that alcoholism and other forms of addictive behavior are a disease. This view is attributed to Jellinek who, in 1960, published *The Disease Concept of Alcoholism*. Most persons now agree that, once substance use proceeds to addiction, a biological component exists. A parallel may be made to depression. An external event may make someone sad or dysphoric. That sadness may worsen into a clinical depression, which has a biological component. Telling a depressed individual to "Stop it" or "Cheer up" is about as useful and empathic as telling an addict to "Just say no." In the case of drug or alcohol addiction, as with depression, medical and mental health intervention is appropriate.

Psychodynamic Model

Psychoanalytic interpretations of substance abuse, based on classical theory, have attributed drug use to oral narcissism, restoration of feelings of omnipotence associated with infantile narcissistic gratification, and regression to oral levels of psychosexual development. One nonspecific concept that may pertain to drug use is Freud's pleasure principle: that we all attempt to avoid pain and increase pleasure. People may use drugs to avoid psychic pain and then continue to use drugs to avoid the pain of withdrawal. Some users, particularly recreational users, may take drugs to increase pleasure temporarily.

Contemporary psychoanalytic practice has moved away from these types of interpretations. Modern practitioners now stress helping the client derive meaning from his or her experiences and to appreciate them as real, important, and distinctly one's own. Stephen A. Mitchell (1993), an author who espouses this view, has written, "What the patient needs is not clarification or insight so much as a sustained experience of being seen, personally engaged, and, basically, valued and cared about" (p. 25).

While practitioners may continue to conceptualize cases in psychodynamic terms, these explanations are often not shared with substance-using clients.

Practitioners may believe that clients are not ready for insight therapy or that psychodynamic descriptions are perceived as negative labels. Many practitioners now believe that individual insight-oriented psychotherapy should begin only after at least one year of other types of treatment, when the client is stabilized, when his or her family and community support systems are mobilized, and when the client is motivated to explore insights about himself or herself. This type of therapy may not be appropriate for many clients.

Integrated Treatment

A consensus has been emerging among practitioners that substance abuse treatment programs require an integration of the various ways of thinking about clients' substance-using behavior. While individual practitioners may still conceptualize the behavior in different ways, for treatment purposes the client is given a holistic and unified view of the problem. An integrated treatment plan then follows from this view. Such treatment may include the following elements:

Elements of Integrated Treatment

- Assessment
- Detoxification
- Medical and psychopharmacological treatments
- Participation in twelve-step programs
- Methadone maintenance if appropriate
- Relapse-prevention training
- Family counseling
- Individual counseling/psychotherapy

Assessment includes evaluation of substance abuse, psychiatric diagnoses, and HIV infection. Detoxification is usually conducted in an inpatient setting but may be done on an outpatient basis depending on the community norms of treatment and available resources. Medical and psychopharmacological treatments are used when appropriate and can be supplemented by enrollment in twelve-step programs. Methadone maintenance for heroin addiction is prescribed when necessary. Other elements of treatment are relapse-prevention training and family and individual counseling or psychotherapy.

Relationships between Substance Abuse and HIV

Because so many people have contracted HIV disease as a result of substance use, it is important that substance abuse counselors learn about HIV and that CMHC staff who are counseling persons with HIV know about substance abuse. We know that body fluids from an infected person transmit the virus and that this may occur when injecting drug users share syringes or "works." Substance use facilitates the spread of HIV infection in the following ways.

Ways That Substance Abuse Facilitates the Spread of HIV

- People who inject drugs and share needles and syringes may exchange HIV-infected blood.
- People who use drugs that weaken their inhibitions and impair their judgment may engage in unsafe sexual practices.
- People may exchange sex for drugs and ignore safer sex practices.
- People infected through injection drug use may sexually transmit HIV to nonusing partners.

Exchange of Body Fluids via Injecting Drugs

Several drugs are administered through needles. The most common is heroin. Cocaine may also be needle-injected. Combinations of heroin and cocaine, called "speedball," are used by some addicts. If a person infected with the virus "shoots up" and then shares the needle with another person, that second person may become infected, because blood from the first person remains in the uncleaned needle and syringe. Addicts are advised not to share needles or syringes. Those who continue to share are urged to clean the needles and syringes with a combination of bleach and water before each use.

Disinhibiting Effects of Drugs

Drug use facilitates the spread of HIV because it can lower a person's inhibitions and impair judgment. A person under the influence of a drug, including alcohol, may unwisely have sex and may fail to take the proper precautions. Suggested safer sex practices for people who use drugs include proper use of a condom or mutual masturbation rather than penetration.

Sex for Drugs and Drug Money

In both urban and rural areas, there are men and women who prostitute for drugs or drug money. The crack cocaine epidemic has fueled prostitution for drugs because users want crack often and because each dose is relatively cheap. Crack addicts often sell themselves cheaply and, at times, are offered additional money if they agree to forego condoms. Unsafe sex, of course, leads to a greater incidence of sexually transmitted diseases, including HIV.

Sexual Transmission from Injecting Drug User (IDU) to Partners

The transmission of HIV through unsafe sexual practices between injecting drug users and their partners is rising. Because there is a large pool of infected substance users, there is an increasing risk of heterosexual transmission. The Surgeon General has estimated that most of the new infections are heterosexually transmitted.

Socioeconomic and Cultural Issues

Screening for Substance Use Regardless of Socioeconomic Factors

The use of drugs and alcohol is not confined to any social, economic, racial, or ethnic class. Many clinicians do not routinely discuss drug use with all of their clients. It is easy to adhere to stereotypes of drug use as dictated by the client's background or class. This is unwise. Drugs may be illegally obtained or prescribed by an inadequately vigilant physician. The most frequently abused drug, alcohol, may be purchased at any liquor store.

Today, because of HIV disease, routine assessment of all clients' substance use and abuse is essential. The following list illustrates the approach that CMHC staff can take in this process.

Screening Clients for Substance Abuse

- Screen every client for substance use and abuse, regardless of background.
- Ask for family history of substance abuse.
- Be suspicious of a history of:
    - Automobile accidents;
    - Revoked or suspended driver's licenses;

–Financial problems;

–Unexplained physical injuries;

–Unexplained job or family problems.

Be vigilant in screening the client's use of tobacco, alcohol, amphetamines, benzodiazepines, and cocaine in its various forms, regardless of the socioeconomic status of the client.

Ask about substance use in the client's family (father, mother, siblings, spouse, partner, and children). A client may be suffering from a spouse's substance-induced brutality or may be forced into unsafe sex. A person who grew up with one or both parents abusing drugs, including alcohol, is at high risk of abuse.

Even though a client may deny drug or alcohol abuse, clinicians should be suspicious if the client has had a driver's license revoked or had a number of accidents. Unexplained money problems despite adequate income, unexplained physical injuries, or job or family problems without adequate explanation may suggest alcohol or other drug abuse.

Sensitivity to Cultural and Subcultural Norms

Our attitudes are communicated to clients, even without the use of words. If we have negative judgments or fail to understand the behavior of clients as symptoms— rather than as completely willful actions—then we cannot hope to provide therapeutic interventions. We need to be aware of several issues involving culture and subculture.

Examples of Cultural Issues That May Affect Care

- Difficulty acknowledging that one cannot handle all stressors
- Mistrust of professional care providers
- Culturally based interpretations of disease and well-being
- Ethnic or racial differences between the therapist and the client
- Language barriers

In cultures where self-sufficiency or privacy are valued, seeking help for mental health problems is difficult. For every one of us, substance user or not, it is extremely difficult to come to a mental health facility and confess to a stranger that one has not been able to prevail over life's stressors. Men, especially, have a difficult time admitting they are only human. Much shame and guilt can be associated with substance use.

Many of our clients may come from communities that perceive medical and mental healthcare providers as unempathic or disrespectful. These communities are suspicious of professional healthcare providers. These issues should be discussed without defensiveness.

Individuals may not ascribe the same sense of importance to their HIV infection as do professional providers. For many persons from lower socioeconomic backgrounds, HIV infection is just one more in a long list of psychosocial stressors. Thus, when a client seems unfazed by an HIV diagnosis, he or she may simply have more immediate and pressing issues. For these clients, poverty, homelessness, malnutrition, neglect and abuse, arrests, and contacts with child welfare agencies may be more pressing than HIV treatment. A nonjudgmental spirit of inquiry about what is blocking compliance with medical treatment may be helpful.

If the therapist is white and is attempting to forge a relationship with a client of color, the issue of cultural differences should be addressed. The therapist is urged to take a stance in which he or she acknowledges the difference, asks the client to share information about his or her life and culture, and encourages the client to explore feelings regarding racial and cultural issues.

Language barriers may create problems between therapists and clients. Wherever possible, clients should be able to speak with someone who shares their language. For example, a CMHC serving Hispanic neighborhoods probably employs Spanish-speaking staff.

Assessment of HIV-Positive Clients with Histories of Substance Use

A thorough assessment is required for HIV-positive clients who are using drugs or who have histories of substance use for several reasons. First, an HIV-positive person has an unpredictable course of illness. Accurate baseline data is necessary to measure changes later. Second, substance users may have both psychiatric and substance abuse diagnoses, which cannot be adequately differentiated without attention and time. Third, the neurological and stress effects of HIV may be additive to create a triple diagnosis: mental disorder, substance abuse, and HIV-related symptoms.

The assessment provides the basis for your decisions about the type of treatment and the level of resources necessary for the client. A thorough assessment should always include the following components:

Components of an Assessment

■ Medical history, including HIV status
■ Client's knowledge and compliance

- Cognitive functioning
- Psychiatric/psychological history
- History of substance use
- Psychosocial/cultural background and support systems

Medical History

A thorough medical history should include the following background information. Is the client HIV-positive and, if so, asymptomatic or symptomatic? Have there been any previous HIV-related conditions and illnesses, including opportunistic infections? What is the client's history of non-HIV substance abuse-related conditions, such as endocarditis, cellulitis, liver problems, or pancreatitis? Does the client have other medical conditions such as diabetes, hypertension, or sickle cell anemia? Ask what medications the client is taking for his or her HIV condition.

Client's Knowledge and Compliance

How accurate is the client's perception of his or her condition? How informed is the client about HIV or substance abuse? Is the client in denial? What is the level of compliance with treatment? What are the possible barriers to following medical regimens (e.g., illiteracy, other learning disability, low IQ, homelessness, lack of medical insurance)?

Cognitive Functioning

Assess cognitive functioning, both premorbid and current. Has there been a deterioration of functioning, either acutely (which requires immediate action) or with slow progression (e.g., dementing process)? Consider neuropsychological assessment and referral for assistance to deal with dementia.

Psychiatric/Psychological History

More than 75 percent of those who use drugs other than alcohol are likely to have a major psychiatric diagnosis. Further, other diagnoses may emerge under the stress of HIV infection. A full history is required to determine premorbid functioning, which may be poor. Mental health interventions should be designed for persons with dual or triple (with HIV) diagnoses.

History of Substance Use

The following issues should be considered by the counselor. He or she should ask at what age the person began to use drugs or alcohol. Use at an early age is indicative of early problems. The counselor should also ask what substances are being used, including the frequency and amount. Polysubstance use is common. The interviewer should ask why these are the substances of choice and what negative effects and consequences the client experiences. The client's readiness for treatment can then be assessed.

Psychosocial/Cultural Background and Support Systems

Assess the psychosocial supports available to the client, including family and community support systems. Will these supports remain through the course of illness? Is there substance abuse or HIV infection among other family members? Has the client experienced losses of loved ones to HIV? How does the client identify himself or herself culturally and in terms of sexual orientation?

Treatment Issues

Integration of Mental Health and Substance Abuse Treatments

Federal policymakers are now encouraging the integration of primary care, substance abuse, and mental health services either at single settings or in linked consortia of community providers. Federal agencies will fund more open competition contracts to provide these integrated services. Meanwhile, studies at sites now providing integrated services are being conducted to determine the cost-effectiveness of such models.

Anecdotal evidence now indicates that higher levels of care are provided in these types of settings. Persons who ordinarily would not seek out services take advantage of integrated services when they are convenient and when providers are nonjudgmental (Kwasnik, Moynihan, & Royle, 1997).

Integrated settings generally are noted for cooperation among psychiatrists, psychologists, social workers, nurses, and others from various disciplines. Many professional disciplines have different presumptions about the cause and treatments of substance abuse. Interdisciplinary teams are often able to avoid hierarchy and appreciate the contributions of the different disciplines. These settings often develop unified treatment plans, based on the biopsychosocial model, which take into account the factors of psychiatric illness, psychological distress, community and culture, and medical aspects of substance abuse, HIV, and other conditions.

In such integrated settings, cases are viewed differently by different practitioners, but the treatment team presents a unified stance, conceptualization, and treatment plan to the client. There is also the opportunity for cross-training, in which practitioners of various disciplines can teach each other. For example, psychiatrists explain psychopharmacology while social workers explain case management. Such a program enriches all practitioners as well as clients.

Case Management Issues

Persons who are HIV-infected require services that are not necessarily included in traditional theoretical frameworks and their associated psychotherapy treatments. In the course of HIV disease, the client is likely to require a therapist who will monitor medical, psychological, and social functioning for signs of deterioration. The therapist will make active interventions that require a range of actions including discussing and overcoming the client's objections to action, mobilizing the client's support systems, and arranging for emergency assistance (Eversole, 1997). Clients also need a case manager who is cognizant of community entitlements and support systems, such as Medicaid, Supplemental Security Income (SSI), home healthcare, and HIV support groups.

While many therapists have avoided involvement with community support services, some providers have realized that the client who may ordinarily avoid counselors may actually approach them with requests for help with entitlements and support services. Counselors can then use such opportunities to address other therapeutic issues.

Use of a Flexible Therapeutic Framework

No single, unbending therapeutic framework is able to serve a client's needs throughout the course of illness (Winiarski, 1991). Immediately after diagnosis, the client may require crisis and family intervention for support. Through the asymptomatic period, the client will benefit from attention to the substance abuse disorder, adherence to medical regimens, and to goals that help to give life meaning. At a later stage of HIV-related illness, the client may require case management and help in obtaining services such as entitlements, home healthcare, and coordination of providers. Service providers' attitudes and abilities, the structure of the clinical setting, and the client's individual requirements are all components of an effective therapeutic contract.

Review Questions

1. What are two ways that drug use facilitates the spread of HIV?

2. Identify some cultural issues that may impede successful engagement of a drug abuser in treatment.

3. What are some of the components of assessing an HIV-infected client with a history of substance abuse?

4. Discuss the relationship between substance abuse and HIV/AIDS.

References and Suggested Readings

Eversole, T. (1997). Psychotherapy and counseling: Bending the frame. In M.G. Winiarski (Ed.), *HIV Mental Health for the 21st Century.* (23–38). New York: New York University Press.

Institute of Medicine. (1990). *Broadening the base of treatment for alcohol problems: Report of a study by a committee of the Institute of Medicine, Division of Mental Health and Behavioral Medicine.* Washington, D.C.: National Academy Press.

Jellinek, E.M. (1960). *The Disease Concept of Alcoholism.* Highland Park, NJ: Hillhouse Press.

Kwasnik, B.C., Moynihan, R.T., & Royle, M.H. (1997). HIV mental health services integrated with medical care. In M.G. Winiarski (Ed.). *HIV Mental Health for the 21st Century.* (209–223). New York: New York University Press.

Marlatt, G.A., & Gordon, J.R. (Eds.) (1985). *Relapse Prevention: Maintenance Strategies in the Treatment of Addictive Behaviors.* New York: Guilford Press.

Miller, W.R., & Rollnick, S. (Eds.) (1991). *Motivational Interviewing: Preparing People to Change Addictive Behavior.* New York: Guilford Press.

Mitchell, S.A. (1993). *Hope and Dread in Psychoanalysis.* New York: Basic Books.

Orford, J. (1985). *Excessive Appetites: A Psychological View of Addictions.* New York: John Wiley & Sons.

Peele, S. (Ed.) (1985). *The Meaning of Addiction: A Compulsive Experience and Its Interpretation.* Lexington, MA: Lexington Books.

Schuckit, M.A. (1989). *Drug and Alcohol Abuse. A Clinical Guide to Diagnosis and Treatment* (3rd ed.). New York: Plenum.

Wallace, B.C. (1991). *Crack Cocaine: A Practical Treatment Approach for the Chemically Dependent.* New York: Bruner/Mazel.

Washton, A.M. (Ed.) (1995). *Psychotherapy and Substance Abuse: A Practitioner's Handbook.* New York: Guilford.

Winiarski, M.G. (Ed.) (1997). *HIV Mental Health for the 21st Century.* New York: New York University Press.

Winiarski, M.G. (1991). *AIDS-Related Psychotherapy.* Elmsford, NY: Pergamon Press. (Now distributed by Allyn & Bacon, Needham Heights, MA).

Appendix

HIV/AIDS Resources

AIDS Hotlines

National AIDS Hotline
Centers for Disease Control and Prevention
(800) 342-2437, TTY (800) 243-7889
(800) 344-7432 (Spanish)

Canadian National AIDS Clearinghouse
Canadian Public Health Association
(613) 725-3434

Alabama	**Alaska**	**Arizona**
(800) 228-0469	(800) 478-2437	(602) 265-3300
Arkansas	**N. California**	**S. California**
(800) 364-2437	(800) 367-2437	(800) 922-2437
Colorado	**Connecticut**	**Delaware**
(800) 252-2437	(800) 203-1234	(800) 422-0429
Washington, D.C.	**Florida**	**Georgia**
(202) 797-3500	(800) 352-2437	(800) 551-2728

Hawaii	Idaho	Illinois
(800) 922-1313	(208) 345-2277	(800) 243-2437
Indiana	Iowa	Kansas
(800) 848-2437	(800) 445-2437	(800) 232-0040
Kentucky	Louisiana	Maine
(800) 654-2437	(800) 922-4379	(800) 851-2437
Maryland	Massachusetts	Michigan
(800) 638-6252	(800) 235-2331	(800) 872-2437
Minnesota	Mississippi	Missouri
(800) 248-2437	(800) 826-2961	(800) 533-2437
Montana	Nebraska	Nevada
(800) 233-6668	(800) 782-2437	(800) 842-2437
New Hampshire	New Jersey	New Mexico
(800) 752-2437	(800) 624-2377	(800) 545-2437
New York	North Carolina	North Dakota
(800) 872-2777	(800) 342-2437	(800) 472-2180
Ohio	Oklahoma	Oregon
(800) 332-2437	(800) 535-2437	(800) 777-2437
Pennsylvania	Puerto Rico	Rhode Island
(800) 662-6080	(809) 765-1010	(800) 726-3010
South Carolina	South Dakota	Tennessee
(800) 322-2437	(800) 592-1861	(800) 525-2437
Texas	Utah	Vermont
(800) 299-2437	(800) 366-2437	(800) 882-2437
Virgin Islands	Virginia	Washington
(809) 773-2437	(800) 533-4148	(800) 272-2437
West Virginia	Wisconsin	Wyoming
(800) 642-8244	(800) 334-2437	(800) 327-3577

Education and Prevention

American Psychological Association
Office on AIDS
750 First St., NE.
Washington, D.C. 20002
(202) 336-6042

The Academy for Educational Development
1875 Connecticut Ave., NW., Suite 900, Washington, D.C. 20009
(202) 884-8000

Office of HIV/AIDS Education
American Red Cross
8111 Gatehouse Rd., Falls Church, VA 22042
(800) 375-2040
http://www.redcross.org/hss/hivaids.html
e-mail: info@usa.redcross.org

Council of State and Territorial Epidemiologists
2872 Woodcock Blvd., Suite 303, Atlanta, GA 30341
(770) 458-3811
e-mail: forr102w@wonder.em.cdc.gov

Gay Men's Health Crisis
119 W. 24th St., New York, NY 10011
(212) 807-6655 (hotline), TTY (212) 645-7470
http://www.gmhc.org

International AIDS Society
PO Box 5619, S-11486 Stockholm, Sweden
011-46-8-612-11-11
http://www.ias.se
e-mail: ias@congrex.se

International Society for HIV/AIDS Education and Prevention
66 Bovet Rd., Suite 270, San Mateo, CA 94402
(415) 573-2385

National AIDS Clearinghouse
Centers for Disease Control and Prevention
U.S. Department of Health and Human Services
PO Box 6003, Rockville, MD 20849
(800) 458-5231 (English and Spanish), TTY (301) 243-7012
http://www.cdcnac.org
e-mail: aidsinfo@cdcnac.org

National Alliance of State and Territorial AIDS Directors
444 N. Capitol St., NW., Suite 706, Washington, D.C. 20001
(202) 434-8090
e-mail: nastad@aol.com

National Association of People With AIDS
1413 K St., NW., 7th Floor, Washington, D.C. 20005
(202) 898-0414, (202) 898-0435 (fax on demand)
http://www.thecure.org
e-mail: napwa@thecure.org

National Coalition of Hispanic Health and Human Services
Organizations, Community HIV and AIDS Technical Assistance
Network
1501 16th St., NW., Washington, D.C. 20036
(202) 387-5000
http://www.cossmho.org
e-mail: cossmho@cossmho.org

National Council of Negro Women
633 Pennsylvania Ave., NW., Washington, D.C. 20004
(202) 737-0120
http://www.ncnw.org

National Hemophilia Foundation, Hemophilia and AIDS/HIV
Network for Dissemination of Information
110 Greene St., SoHo Bld., Suite 303, New York, NY 10012
(800) 424-2634
http://www.infonhf.org

National Minority AIDS Council
300 I St., NE., Suite 400, Washington, D.C. 20002
(202) 483-6622
http://www.thebody.com/nmac/nmacpage.html

National Native American AIDS Prevention Center
3515 Grand Ave., Suite 100, Oakland, CA 94610
(800) 283-2437, (800) 283-6880 (fax on demand)
e-mail: nnaapc@aol.com

National Pediatric and Family HIV Resource Center
15 S. 9th St., Newark, NJ 07107
(800) 362-0071
http://www.wdcnet.com/PedsAIDS/
e-mail: nphrc@daiid.umdnj.edu

National Resource Center on Women and AIDS
Center for Women Policy Studies
1211 Connecticut Ave., NW., Suite 312, Washington, D.C. 20036
(202) 872-1770
e-mail: hn4066@handsnet.org

National Task Force on AIDS Prevention
973 Market St., Suite 600, San Francisco, CA 94103
(415) 356-8100
e-mail: ntsap@aol.com

United States–Mexico Border Health Association
6006 North Mesa St., Suite 600, El Paso, TX 79912
(915) 581-6648
e-mail: usmbha@aol.com

USF Center For HIV Education and Research
University of South Florida
13301 Bruce B. Downs Blvd., Tampa, FL 33612
(813) 974-4430
http://www.fmhi.usf.edu/aidscenter.html
e-mail: hivcntr@fmhi.usf.edu

Epidemiology

National Center for Health Statistics
Centers for Disease Control and Prevention
U.S. Department of Health and Human Services
6525 Belcrest Rd., Hyattsville, MD 20782
(301) 436-8500
http://www.cdc.gov/nchswww/nchshome.htm

National Center for HIV, STD, and TB Prevention
Centers for Disease Control and Prevention
U.S. Department of Health and Human Services
1600 Clifton Road, NE., Atlanta, GA 30333
(404) 639-2076
(404) 639-2076 (statistical information line—recorded)
(800) 458-5231 (reference specialist)
http://www.cdc.gov/nchstp/od/nchstp.html
e-mail: NCHSTP@cpsod1.em.cdc.gov

Pan American Health Organization
Regional Office of the World Health Organization
525 23rd St., NW., Washington, D.C. 20037
(202) 974-3000
http://www.paho.org

Political, Social, Legal

AIDS Action Council
1875 Connecticut Ave., NW., Suite 700, Washington, D.C. 20009
(202) 986-1300
http://www.thebody.com/aac/aacpage.html
e-mail: nh3384@handsnet.org

AIDS Coalition to Unleash Power, New York
332 Bleeker St., Suite G5, New York, NY 10014
(212) 564-2437
http://www.actupny.org
e-mail: actupny@panix.com

AIDS National Interfaith Network
1400 I St., NW., Suite 1220, Washington, D.C. 20005
(800) 288-9619
http://www.thebody.com/anin/aninpage.html

American Psychological Association
Public Interest Directorate, Office on AIDS
750 First St., NE., Washington, D.C. 20002
(202) 336-6042
http://www.apa.org
e-mail: publicinterest@apa.org

Americans for a Sound AIDS/HIV Policy
PO Box 17433, Washington, D.C. 20041
(703) 471-7350

Association of Nurses in AIDS Care
1555 Connecticut Ave., NW., Suite 200, Washington, D.C. 20036
(202) 462-1038, (202) 234-3587 (fax on demand)
http://www.mc.vanderbilt.edu/adl/pathfinders/missions/anac.html
e-mail: aidsnurse@apl.com

International Association of Physicians in AIDS Care
225 W. Washington St., Suite 2200, Chicago, IL 60608
(312) 527-2025
http://www.iapac.org/index.html
e-mail: iapac@iapac.org

National Association of Community Health Centers
1330 New Hampshire Ave., NW., Washington, D.C. 20036
(202) 659-8008

National Community Mental Healthcare Council
12300 Twinbrook Parkway, Suite 320, Rockville, MD 20852
(301) 984-6200

National Leadership Coalition on AIDS
1400 I St., NW., Suite 1220, Washington, D.C. 20005
(202) 408-4848

Pediatric AIDS Foundation
1311 Colorado Ave, Santa Monica, CA 90404
(310) 395-9051

People with AIDS Coalition
50 W. 17th St., 8th Floor, New York, NY 10011
(212) 532-0290, (800) 828-3280 (hotline)

Project Inform
1965 Market St., Suite 220, San Francisco, CA 94103
(800) 822-7422
http://www.projinf.org

Research and Treatment

AIDS Clinical Trials Information Service
PO Box 6421, Rockville, MD 20849
(800) 874-2572 (English and Spanish), TTY (800) 243-7012
(301) 217-0023 (international)
http://www.actis.org
e-mail: actis@cdcnac.org

American Foundation for AIDS Research
1828 L St., NW., Suite 802, Washington, D.C. 20036
(202) 331-8600
e-mail: asmfardc@aol.com

HIV/AIDS Treatment Information Service
PO Box 6303, Rockville, MD 20849
(800) 448-0440, TTY (800) 243-7012
(301) 217-0023 (international)
http://www.hivatis.org
e-mail: atis@cdcnac.org

International AIDS Society for Natural and Traditional Medicines, Natural, Alternative, Traditional and Complementary Therapies Caucus
PO Box 21735, Washington, D.C. 20009
(202) 234-9632
e-mail: cntm@aol.com

National HIV Telephone Consultation Service—Warm Line
AIDS Education and Training Centers Health Resources and Service Administration
(800) 933-3413 7:50 am–5:00 pm PST Monday–Friday
http://itsa.ucsf.edu/~libbys/

National Institutes of Health
6003 Executive Blvd., Room 2A07, Bethesda, MD 20892
(301) 496-4000
http://www.nih.gov
e-mail: nihinfo@od31tm1.od.nih.gov

Support Services

AIDS Memorial Quilt
NAMES Project Foundation
310 Townsend, Suite 310, San Francisco, CA 94107
(415) 882-5500
http://www.aidsquilt.org
e-mail: info@aidsquilt.org

Alliance AIDS Housing Network
National Alliance to End Homelessness
1518 K St., NW., Suite 206, Washington, D.C. 20005
(202) 638-1526
e-mail: naeh@ari.net

AIDS Resource Committee
National Hospice Organization
1901 N. Moore St., Suite 901, Arlington, VA 22209
(800) 658-8898
http://www.nho.org
e-mail: drsnho@cais.com

Index

Page numbers in *italics* denote figures; those followed by "t" denote tables.